ADHD LIFE SKILLS 101:

A COMPREHENSIVE GUIDE FOR PARENTAL INSIGHT, IMPROVED EMOTIONAL SUPPORT, PROFESSIONAL DEVELOPMENT FOR THERAPISTS, AND UNDERSTANDING ADHD

JAMAAL SIMMONS, LCSW-C

In loving memory and honor of my Uncle Stan, my cousin Jermaine (aka Dirty Money), my mother in Law Patricia Wilson, and my brother Dylan Rodriguez.

FORWARD FROM TERRI E. JOHNSON:

When Jamaal Simmons first approached me with the idea for ADHD Life Skills 101, I knew immediately that this book would be something special. Jamaal is not just an author; he is a mentee, a friend, and a shining example of how ADHD, when understood and harnessed, can become a superpower.

As someone who has navigated the complexities of ADHD since childhood, I have experienced firsthand the challenges and triumphs that come with this disorder. Growing up, I often felt like I was living in a world that moved at a different pace than I did—where distractions were a constant companion, focus felt like a fleeting dream, and the expectations of school and social environments often left me feeling overwhelmed.

For many years, I struggled to understand myself, often feeling isolated and frustrated. The symptoms of ADHD—impulsivity, inattention, and hyperactivity—colored my experiences, making it difficult to keep up with peers and meet the expectations of teachers and family. I remember moments of despair, thinking that I would never find my footing in a world that seemed to demand constant attention and organization.

However, my journey took a positive turn when I began exploring treatment options. With the support of healthcare professionals, I found a medication that worked for me. It was as if a fog had lifted; I could finally see the world clearly and engage with it in a meaningful way. The medication did not change who I am but rather helped me harness my strengths while managing the challenges of ADHD.

Through this journey, I learned that success is not solely defined by traditional measures. It is about finding what works for you and embracing your unique path. I discovered that my creativity, energy, and ability to think outside the box—traits often linked to ADHD—could be powerful assets when channeled effectively.

As an adult, I have built a fulfilling life, both personally and professionally. I have learned to advocate for myself, seek support when needed, and celebrate my achievements, no matter how small they may seem. My experiences have equipped me with resilience and empathy, allowing me to connect with others who face similar struggles.

In sharing my story, I hope to shed light on the realities of living with ADHD and to inspire those who may feel lost in their own journeys. It is essential to remember that while ADHD presents challenges, it also offers unique strengths that can lead to incredible accomplishments. With the right support and understanding, we can navigate the complexities of this disorder and thrive in our own extraordinary ways.

Thank you for joining me in this exploration of ADHD, where we will delve deeper into its intricacies, share insights, and foster a community of understanding and support. Together, we can turn the page on stigma and celebrate the diverse experiences of those living with ADHD.

Terri E. Johnson, cctp-II, lcadc, acsw, lcsw-c

Clinical Social Worker

Author of Body Saftey Zones (BSZ)

Link to Terri E. Johnson's Children's Book:

https://www.etsy.com/shop/PersistenceistheWAY

CONTENTS

INTRODUCTION

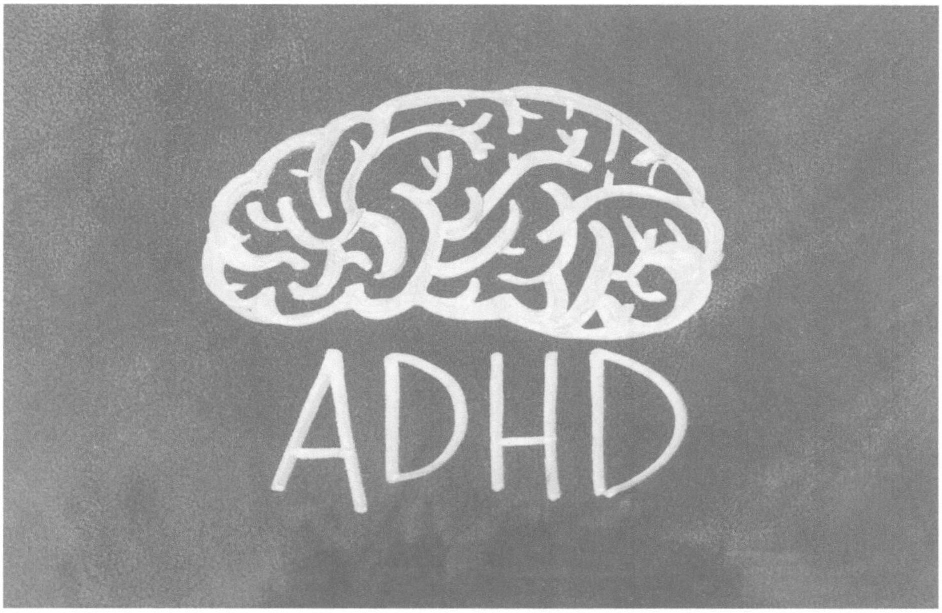

As a clinical therapist with ADHD as an adult, I know firsthand the exhilaration and exhaustion that come with having a mind that never seems to slow down. I remember the day I sat in my office, staring at a pile of unfinished paperwork, feeling utterly overwhelmed. Suddenly, a client burst in, excited to share a breakthrough they had during our last session. At that moment, I realized that my ability to think quickly and connect ideas had allowed me to make a real difference in someone's life. This epiphany sparked my journey to understand and embrace my ADHD, ultimately leading me to write this book.

"ADHD Life Skills 101" is your stress-free guide to understanding and optimizing your ADHD potential. This book aims to transform your perception of ADHD from a limitation to an incredible asset that can enhance your personal growth. By exploring the unique challenges and strengths of adult ADHD, you'll discover how to harness your natural creativity, innovation, and resilience.

Many people think of ADHD as a childhood disorder, but it affects millions of adults worldwide. Adult ADHD can manifest differently, impacting relationships, work performance, and overall well-being. Despite its prevalence, there are still many misconceptions surrounding adult ADHD. This book seeks to dispel those myths and provide you with a clear understanding of what it means to live with ADHD as an adult.

What sets this book apart is its holistic approach, combining practical strategies with interactive elements designed specifically for adults with ADHD. You'll find reflective exercises and self-assessment tools that help you gain insight into your unique ADHD experience. The book also integrates wellness practices, such as nutrition advice, exercise recommendations, and mindfulness techniques, recognizing the importance of self-care in managing ADHD symptoms.

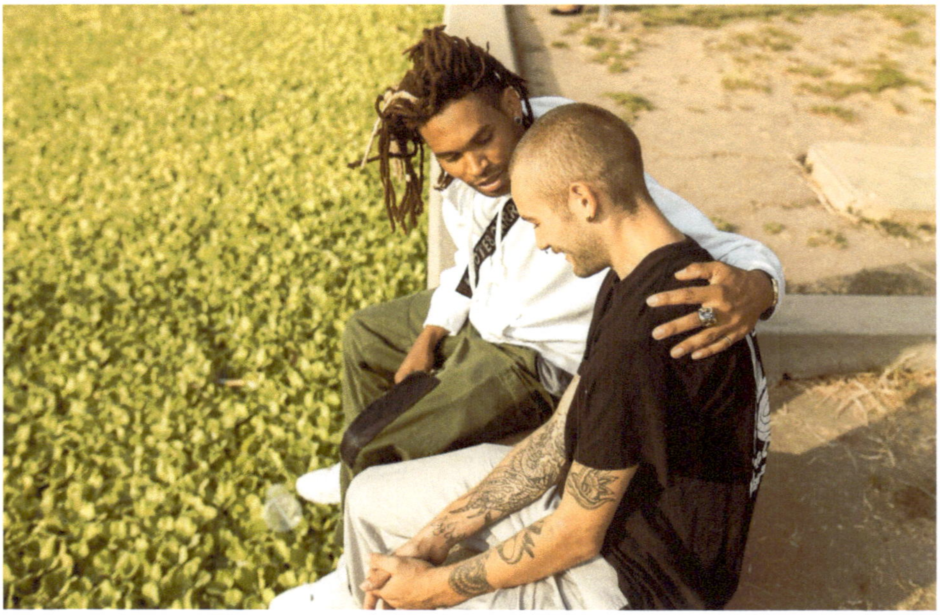

Throughout this journey, it's crucial to remember that you're not alone. ADHD affects people from all walks of life, and cultural differences can shape how it is perceived and managed. By fostering a sense of community and inclusion, this book aims to help you feel understood and supported as you navigate your ADHD journey.

As you progress through the chapters, you'll explore key themes such as time management, emotional regulation, relationship building, and career development. Each section is designed to build upon the last, providing you with a comprehensive toolkit for success. The ADHD-friendly structure and visual layout—complete with clear headings, bullet points, and colorful illustrations—will keep you engaged and focused.

But this book is more than just a passive read – it's an interactive experience. I encourage you to participate actively in the exercises, reflect on your thoughts and feelings, and apply the strategies to your daily life. By engaging with the material, you'll not only gain a deeper understanding of your ADHD but also develop the skills to thrive in all aspects of your life.

As we embark on this journey together, I want to leave you with a final thought: embracing your ADHD is an act of self-love and empowerment. By learning to appreciate and work with your unique brain wiring, you open yourself to a world of possibilities. So, let's dive in and discover how to make your ADHD work for you, not against you. Together, we'll unlock your full potential and create a life that truly fulfills you.

CHAPTER 1

UNDERSTANDING YOUR ADHD

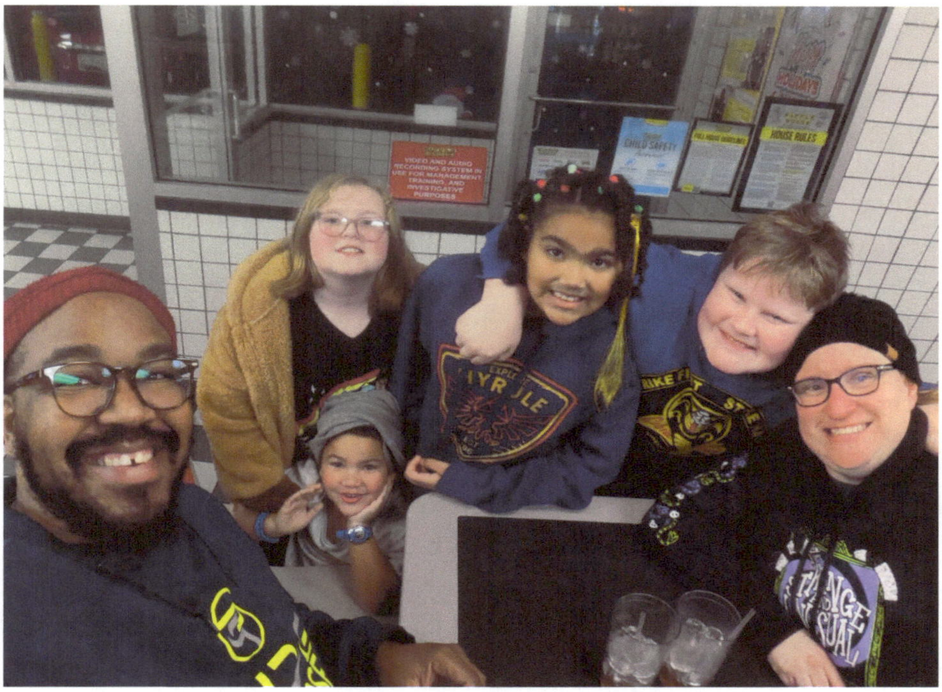

Waffle House - left to right (myself, Cat, Henry, Gloria, JJ, Michelle)

THERE WAS A TIME, not too long ago, when I perceived my ADHD as a relentless storm, constantly churning up chaos in my life. I was sitting in a Waffle House, trying to order food with my family and then-girlfriend—now my fiancée, Michelle—along with my two kids and her two kids. But my mind was racing through a dozen unrelated thoughts. Despite the noise and distractions, an unexpected idea surfaced—a creative solution to a problem I'd been wrestling with for weeks. It struck me then that my ADHD was not just turbulence; it was also the gust that propelled me forward, guiding me to unexpected shores of creativity and insight. That moment, along with trying out Adderall, was a catalyst in my understanding of ADHD, prompting a shift in perspective that I hope to share with you in this chapter.

EMBRACING NEURODIVERSITY

Neurodiversity is a term that has gained traction over the past few decades. It was coined by sociologist Judy Singer to describe the diversity of human brains and the different ways they function. It suggests that conditions like ADHD, autism, dyslexia, and others aren't just disorders but variations in the human genome that offer unique strengths and perspectives. Understanding ADHD through the lens of neurodiversity reframes it from a deficit to a different way of experiencing the world. This perspective emphasizes that everyone, regardless of cognitive function, has something valuable to contribute. Neurodiversity isn't about defining some people as "normal" and others as "abnormal." Instead, it celebrates the spectrum of human thought and recognizes that differences can lead to innovation and progress. By shifting our focus from deficits to diversity, we see ADHD not as a flaw but as a unique cognitive profile that can drive creativity and problem-solving.

Cultural perspectives on ADHD vary widely, affecting how it's perceived and managed. In Western cultures, there's often an emphasis on diagnosis and treatment, viewing ADHD through a medical lens. In contrast, some Eastern cultures may see ADHD as less of a medical issue and more as a behavioral or character trait, sometimes leading to stigma or misunderstanding. These cultural differences shape how individuals with ADHD are supported—or not—by their communities. In some cultures, the myths surrounding ADHD can create barriers to understanding and acceptance. For instance, the idea that ADHD is merely an excuse for laziness or poor behavior is a misconception that persists in various societies. Recognizing these cultural nuances is crucial in fostering a more inclusive environment where all neurodiverse individuals feel valued and understood.

The strengths of a neurodiverse mind are numerous and profound. Individuals with ADHD often excel in pattern recognition, seeing connections and solutions that might elude others. This ability can lead to innovative approaches in fields like art, science, and business. Hyperfocus—one of the more intriguing aspects of ADHD—allows for intense concentration on tasks of interest, leading to deep dives into subjects and often resulting in groundbreaking discoveries or creations. Moreover, the creativity and out-of-the-box thinking associated with ADHD are invaluable in environments that prize innovation and adaptability. These strengths challenge the traditional narratives that have long stigmatized ADHD, highlighting instead the potential for greatness and achievement.

Creating a neurodiverse-friendly environment starts with acknowledging and valuing these strengths. Flexible work environments, for example, can accommodate the unique needs of those with ADHD, allowing them to thrive. This might mean providing options for remote work, flexible hours, or quiet spaces to minimize distractions. Encouraging diverse teamwork approaches is another critical strategy. By assembling teams with varied cognitive profiles, organizations can benefit from a broader range of ideas and solutions. Embracing neurodiversity in this way not only supports individuals with ADHD but also enriches the collective creativity and productivity of any group.

Reflective Exercise: Identifying Your Unique Strengths

Take a moment to reflect on your experiences with ADHD. What are some of the unique strengths you've discovered along the way? Consider how these strengths have helped you in different aspects of your life—whether at work, in relationships, or in personal pursuits. Write down a few examples and think about how you can leverage these strengths moving forward. Recognizing and embracing your unique abilities is the first step toward transforming ADHD into a powerful asset.

DECODING ADHD SYMPTOMS

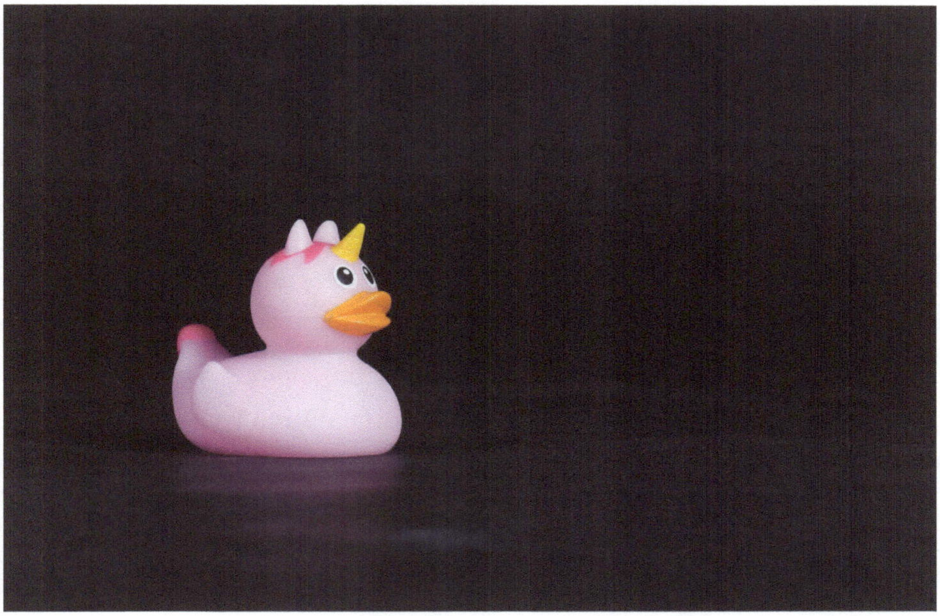

ADHD in adults can be a complex tapestry of symptoms that weave through daily life, often catching us off guard. One of the most pervasive symptoms is inattention, which can feel like trying to hold onto water with open hands. You sit down to tackle a work project, determined to make progress, but your mind wanders—pulled in by the notifications on your phone, the chatter of nearby conversations, or even your own thoughts bouncing around like in *Sonic pinball* while trying to beat the boss. This distractibility can make it challenging to maintain focus, leading to tasks that take longer than they should and resulting in a frustrating cycle of unfinished projects.

On the flip side, hyperactivity might not always manifest as physical restlessness in adults. Instead, it can be a mental restlessness that fuels impulsivity—prompting quick decisions without weighing the consequences or shifting from one task to another without completion. This can lead to impulsive purchases, blurting out thoughts without a filter, or diving headfirst into new projects before finishing existing ones.

Variability in ADHD symptoms means that no two people experience it the same way. Gender differences further complicate this picture, as women with ADHD often present more inattentive symptoms, while men may exhibit more hyperactive-impulsive behaviors. This disparity can lead to different challenges and coping strategies. For instance, a woman might struggle with organizing her daily tasks due to inattentiveness, while a man might find it difficult to control impulsive reactions in social or work settings.

Beyond gender, ADHD presents in different forms—some may experience it predominantly as inattentive ADHD, where focus is the main issue, while others might have hyperactive-impulsive ADHD, characterized by higher energy levels and impulsivity. Still, others might have a combined type, experiencing both sets of symptoms. This variability means that understanding one's unique ADHD profile is crucial for managing it effectively.

The impact of these symptoms on daily life can be profound, often manifesting in the workplace where maintaining focus is critical. For many adults with ADHD, staying on task can feel like an uphill battle, with distractions lurking at every corner. This can lead to missed deadlines, incomplete work, or the need for constant reminders, creating stress and anxiety. Similarly, organizing tasks can be daunting, as the ADHD mind may struggle with prioritizing what needs to be done first, leading to a chaotic approach where urgent tasks are mixed with less important ones. This disorganization can spill over into home life, resulting in cluttered spaces and forgotten commitments.

Time management is another major hurdle, with the ADHD brain often losing track of time—whether due to hyperfocus on a particular task or simply the inability to gauge how long something will take. This can result in chronic tardiness or the feeling of always being behind schedule, affecting both personal and professional relationships.

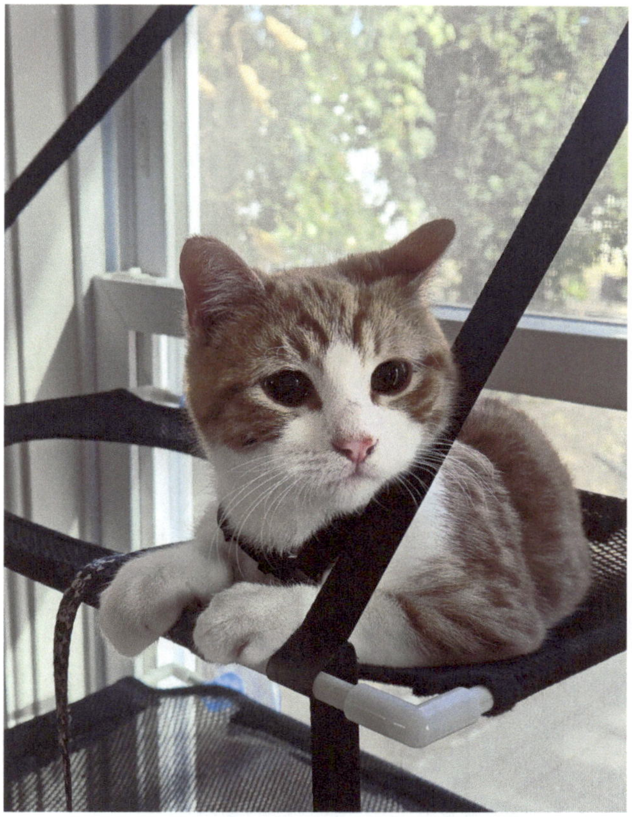

Our new Kitten Milo: the newest employee of Simmons Mental Health LLC

Addressing misconceptions is vital to truly understanding ADHD. Many people still believe that ADHD is just an excuse for laziness or a lack of discipline—a myth that can undermine the self-esteem of those living with it. In reality, ADHD is a neurological condition that affects brain chemistry and function, making certain tasks genuinely more challenging.

Another persistent myth is that ADHD only affects children. While it's true that ADHD is often diagnosed in childhood, many individuals continue to experience symptoms into adulthood, affecting their daily lives in various ways. Recognizing these realities helps dismantle the stigma and encourages a more empathetic understanding of what living with ADHD entails.

Interactive Element: Symptom Self-Assessment

Take a moment to reflect on your own experiences with ADHD symptoms. How do inattention and distractibility show up in your daily life? Do you notice patterns in your hyperactivity or impulsivity? Consider keeping a journal for a week, noting when and how these symptoms appear. This self-assessment can provide valuable insights into your unique ADHD profile, helping you identify areas to focus on for improvement and management. Understanding your symptoms is a powerful step towards navigating the challenges they present.

ADHD AND CREATIVITY: UNLEASHING INNOVATIVE POTENTIAL

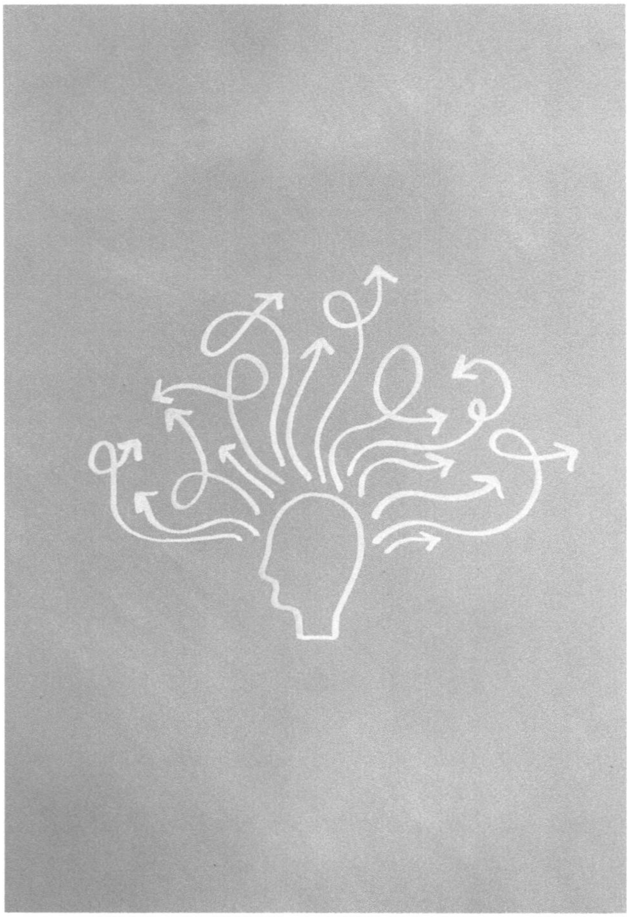

Reflecting on the natural connection between ADHD and creativity, my thoughts drift to an inspiring afternoon at an art gallery with a friend. As we meandered among the artworks, my mind ignited with ideas for a novel project, each piece of art acting as a catalyst for a flurry of interconnected thoughts. This moment epitomizes the unique relationship between ADHD and creativity. Individuals with ADHD are naturally inclined toward divergent thinking—the ability to spawn multiple ideas or solutions from a single point of inspiration. This skill is helpful in my therapy sessions. Our cognitive agility opens up pathways that initially seem disparate yet often lead to revolutionary discoveries. In a society that predominantly appreciates linear and traditional problem-solving, possessing a mind that thrives on diverse and innovative thinking is an invaluable strength.

The spontaneity that comes with ADHD can be a double-edged sword. On one hand, it leads to a constant flow of ideas and an innate ability to think on our feet. On the other, it can sometimes result in a lack of focus or follow-through. But when channeled effectively, this spontaneity can fuel creative processes in remarkable ways. Take the case of Thomas Edison, whose tenacity and innovative spirit led to the invention of the light bulb and countless other devices. Edison's approach was characterized by trial and error—a method that resonates with the ADHD tendency to experiment and iterate until a solution emerges. Similarly, Leonardo da Vinci, with his insatiable curiosity and diverse interests, exemplified the ADHD mind's ability to juggle multiple passions and pursuits. His notebooks reveal a whirlwind of ideas, sketches, and observations—a testament to the creative potential inherent in ADHD.

To harness these creative bursts effectively, it's helpful to employ strategies that provide structure while allowing for flexibility. Structured brainstorming sessions, where ideas are encouraged without judgment, can be immensely productive. During these sessions, you might find that one idea sparks another, leading to a cascade of inspiration. Using mind maps can also be a valuable tool, helping to organize thoughts visually and see connections that might not be apparent in a linear list. By laying out ideas in a web-like format, you can explore different paths and possibilities, giving shape to the creative chaos. Additionally, time-blocking creative work allows you to dedicate specific periods to deep thinking and experimentation, ensuring that creativity doesn't get lost amid daily distractions.

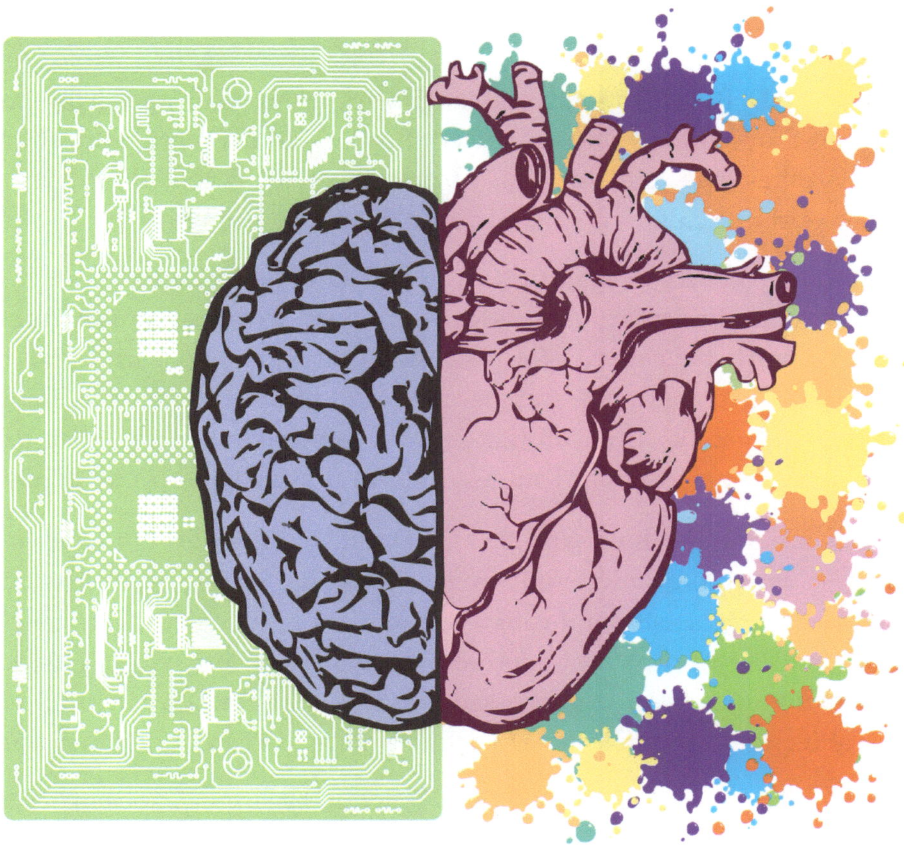

Balancing creativity with practicality is crucial for turning ideas into reality. It starts with setting achievable creative goals that align with your broader objectives. Rather than setting out to complete a massive project all at once, break it down into smaller, manageable tasks that can be tackled incrementally. This approach not only makes the process less daunting but also provides a sense of accomplishment at each step.

Integrating creativity into everyday tasks is another effective strategy. Whether it's finding a new way to tackle a routine chore or approaching a work project with fresh eyes, infusing creativity into daily life can lead to innovative solutions and increased satisfaction. The key is to remain open to new possibilities while maintaining a focus on practical outcomes.

Interactive Element: Channeling Your Creativity

Take some time to engage in a structured brainstorming session. Choose a topic or challenge you're passionate about and set a timer for 20 minutes. Let your ideas flow freely without censoring or judging them. When the timer goes off, review what you've written and use a mind map to explore connections and organize your thoughts. Identify a few key ideas that resonate with you and consider how you might develop them further. By giving yourself the space to explore and structure your creativity, you can transform spontaneous bursts of inspiration into actionable plans.

THE POSITIVE POWER OF ADHD

When we talk about ADHD, it's easy to get caught up in the challenges—the impulsivity, the distractions, the constant battle to stay organized. But let's take a moment to shift the spotlight and illuminate the other side, the side that's brimming with potential and untapped power. ADHD isn't just a set of difficulties; it's a wellspring of unique strengths.

One such strength is resilience. Those of us with ADHD often find ourselves in scenarios that require quick thinking and adaptation. This constant need to adjust and manage life's unpredictability builds a remarkable capacity for resilience. Over time, we learn to bounce back from setbacks, approach problems with new perspectives, and find solutions where others might see only obstacles. This adaptability is a skill that many people spend years trying to develop, and it's something that can propel us toward success in both personal and professional spheres.

High energy levels are another hallmark of ADHD, and while they can sometimes feel overwhelming, they also provide a unique advantage. This energy can be channeled into passion projects, fueling the drive to see them through to completion. It enables us to take on tasks with enthusiasm, often leading to bursts of productivity that catch others off guard. Think about those moments when you've been so engrossed in a task that hours fly by without notice. That is ADHD energy at its finest, propelling us to achieve more than we sometimes think possible.

The world is full of success stories from individuals who have embraced their ADHD traits and turned them into assets. Entrepreneurs are prime examples. Take David Neeleman, the founder of JetBlue Airways, who credits his ADHD with giving him the creativity and out-of-the-box thinking necessary to revolutionize air travel. Or Ingvar Kamprad, the mind behind IKEA, who used his ADHD-driven creativity to design furniture that is both functional and affordable. These individuals didn't see ADHD as a limitation; they saw it as a superpower that set them apart, allowing them to innovate and succeed in ways others couldn't.

The arts are another realm where ADHD shines brightly. Artists and innovators often speak about their ADHD as a source of inspiration. The ability to think divergently—to see the world not as it is but as it could be—is a gift that can lead to groundbreaking work. The arts thrive on fresh perspectives and novel ideas, both of which are abundant in the ADHD mind. Whether it's a painter experimenting with new techniques or a musician composing an unexpected harmony, ADHD can drive creativity in powerful ways.

Building confidence is crucial for those with ADHD, as years of feeling misunderstood or underestimated can erode self-esteem. Celebrating small victories is a great way to start. Each task completed and goal achieved, no matter how minor, is a step forward and deserves recognition. Developing a growth mindset—where we focus on progress and learning rather than perfection—can also bolster confidence. It encourages us to see mistakes as opportunities for growth rather than failures, fostering a more positive self-image.

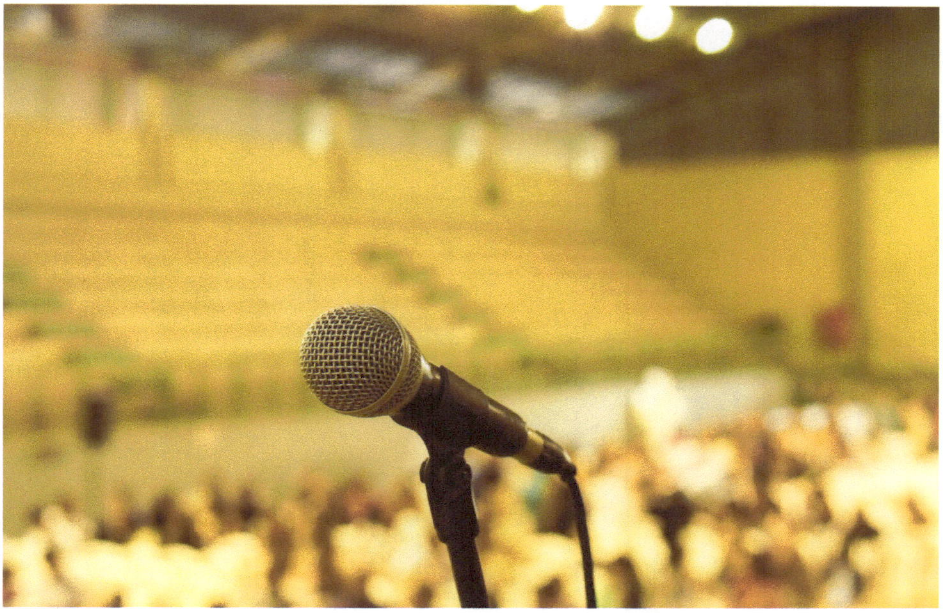

Advocacy and awareness play pivotal roles in transforming public perception of ADHD. By promoting ADHD awareness campaigns, we can educate others about the strengths and challenges associated with the condition, breaking down stigma and fostering understanding. Engaging in community support groups provides a platform for sharing experiences and advice, creating a sense of belonging and empowerment among individuals with ADHD. These groups are invaluable for advocacy, as they offer collective voices that can push for policy changes and greater acceptance.

As we move forward, it's important to remember that ADHD is not something to be hidden or ashamed of. It's a part of who we are—a part that brings with it the potential for incredible achievements and personal growth. By reframing ADHD as a strength, we can unlock possibilities that go beyond what we might have thought possible. Let's embrace this perspective, not just for ourselves but for everyone who sees the world through the ADHD lens.

The power of ADHD lies in its ability to defy conventions and inspire innovation, and by recognizing this, we can transform lives—our own included.

CHAPTER 2
MASTERING TIME MANAGEMENT

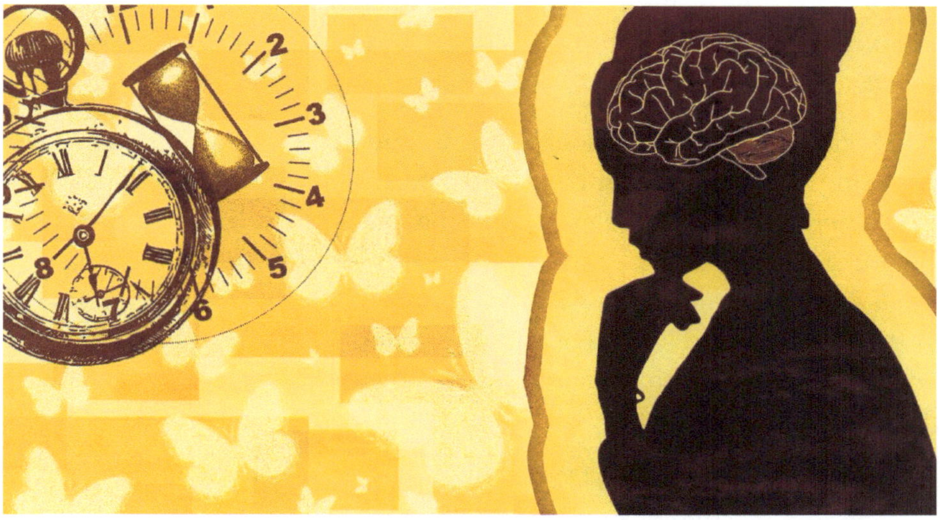

TIME MANAGEMENT HAS ALWAYS BEEN one of those elusive skills that seem to slip through my fingers—much like trying to catch the wind. I remember a particularly chaotic day when I had multiple deadlines looming, each demanding my attention like a chorus of clashing cymbals. My mind was a whirlwind of distractions, and I felt paralyzed by the sheer volume of tasks. It was then that I stumbled upon the Pomodoro Technique, a simple and underrated yet effective method that transformed the way I approached my work. Developed by Francesco Cirillo in the late 1980s, it involves breaking tasks into 25-minute focused sessions called Pomodoros, with short breaks in between. This method not only helped me regain control over my schedule but also revealed a new way of working that aligned perfectly with the ADHD brain's need for structure and variety.

The origins of the Pomodoro Technique are quite straightforward, yet its simplicity is what makes it so powerful. Cirillo named the method after the Italian word for tomato, inspired by the tomato-shaped kitchen timer he used during his university days to track his work sessions. The technique's genius lies in its ability to turn overwhelming tasks into manageable chunks—a concept that resonates deeply with those of us who struggle with time perception and task management. For individuals with ADHD, this approach offers a structured framework that fosters focus and reduces the anxiety of facing seemingly insurmountable tasks. By breaking down work into 25-minute sprints, followed by five-minute breaks, the technique mirrors the natural ebb and flow of attention, making it an ideal tool for enhancing productivity.

Implementing the Pomodoro Technique is surprisingly easy, and its impact can be felt almost immediately. Start by choosing a task you need to tackle, whether it's writing a report, organizing your workspace, or even sorting through emails. Set a timer for 25 minutes and immerse yourself in the task, allowing nothing to distract you. When the timer rings, take a short five-minute break to recharge—stretch your legs, grab a drink, or simply breathe. After completing four Pomodoros, reward yourself with a longer break—anywhere from 15 to 30 minutes—to give your mind a chance to rest and reset. This cycle not only helps maintain focus but also prevents burnout, a common pitfall for those with ADHD who often hyperfocus for extended periods without taking breaks.

Maximizing productivity with the Pomodoro Technique involves more than just setting a timer. It's about prioritizing tasks and recognizing when adjustments are needed. At the start of each session, take a moment to identify the most pressing tasks—those that require immediate attention or have looming deadlines. By concentrating on these priorities, you ensure that the most critical work gets done during your peak focus times. Be mindful of your energy levels and adjust the session lengths if necessary. For some, 25 minutes might be too short or too long, and that's okay. The key is finding a rhythm and flow that works for you, allowing you to maintain focus without feeling overwhelmed.

One of the most valuable aspects of the Pomodoro Technique is its ability to track progress and highlight areas for improvement. Keeping a journal of completed Pomodoros can provide insights into your work habits and reveal patterns you might not have noticed before. Are there certain times of day when you're more productive? Do specific tasks consistently take longer than expected? This awareness allows you to make informed adjustments, such as reallocating tasks to different times or breaking them down further. By identifying these patterns, you can tailor your approach to suit your unique needs, ultimately leading to a more efficient and satisfying workflow.

Reflective Exercise: Your Pomodoro Journal

To get started with the Pomodoro Technique, consider keeping a simple journal to track your sessions. Note down the task you're working on, the number of pomodoros completed, and any observations about your focus and productivity. Over time, review your entries to identify trends and areas for adjustment. This small step can lead to significant improvements in how you manage your time and tasks, helping you harness the full potential of the Pomodoro Technique.

VISUAL PLANNERS: SEEING YOUR DAY AT A GLANCE

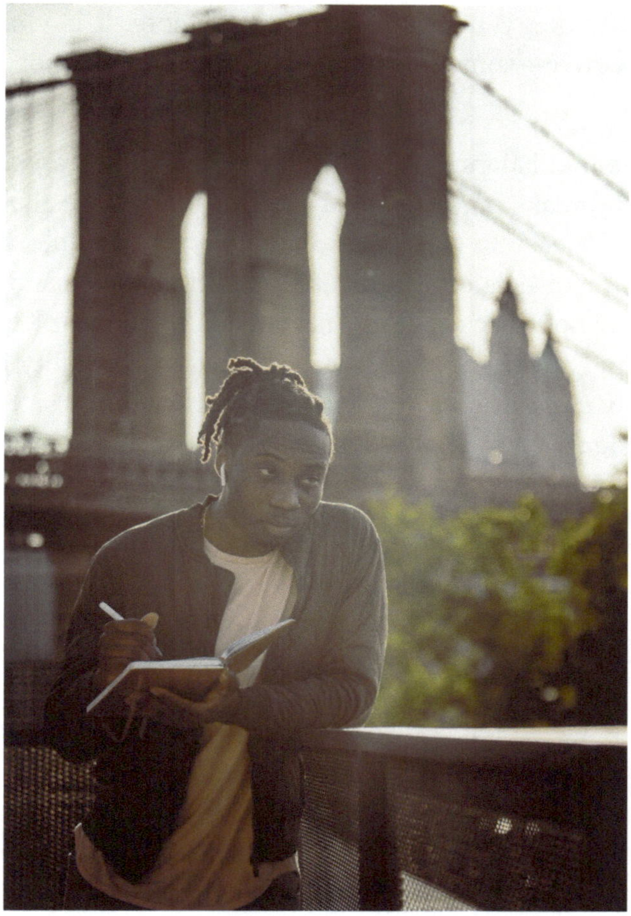

Visual planners have a transformative power that can make a chaotic day feel manageable. For someone with ADHD, the world often moves at a dizzying pace, with thoughts and tasks swirling like leaves caught in a gust of wind. Visual planners offer a way to capture those thoughts and tasks, pinning them down in a manner that's both orderly and accessible. The use of visual cues like color coding and symbols can enhance focus, turning an overwhelming list of responsibilities into a clear path forward. By simplifying tasks and breaking them into manageable segments, visual planners help reduce the sense of being overwhelmed. They transform a tangled web of to-dos into a series of achievable goals, allowing you to see not just the demands of the day but also the opportunities for accomplishment.

Choosing the right planner is a personal journey of discovery. It's about finding a tool that aligns with your preferences and the way your brain processes information. Some people thrive with digital planners, enjoying the flexibility and integration they offer across devices. Others, including myself, prefer the tactile experience of a paper planner, where the act of writing can solidify intentions and keep distractions at bay. Consider what features are most important to you. Color coding can help prioritize and categorize tasks, while time blocks offer a visual representation of how your day is structured. A planner that allows for customization, with sections for notes, goals, and reflections, can provide the structure you need while accommodating the fluidity of daily life. Whatever format you choose, it is vital to find a planner that feels intuitive and supportive—something that will be your ally, not an additional source of stress.

Creating a daily schedule that balances flexibility with structure is an art form in itself. Start by allocating time for work, breaks, and personal activities, ensuring that you don't neglect one area in favor of another. It's easy to let work dominate your schedule, but carving out time for relaxation and personal interests is crucial for maintaining balance and well-being. Set realistic goals for each day, recognizing that not every task needs to be completed right away. Prioritize what's most important and allow space for the unexpected. Flexibility is vital, especially when life's curveballs inevitably come your way. A well-crafted schedule isn't a rigid set of rules but a guide that helps you navigate your day with intention and focus.

Regular reviews of your planner are essential for maintaining its effectiveness. Set aside time each week to assess how well your schedule is working. Are you consistently meeting your goals, or do certain tasks keep getting pushed to the next day? Reflect on your accomplishments and any setbacks, and use these insights to adjust your approach. Perhaps certain tasks need more time than you've allotted, or maybe your priorities have shifted. These weekly check-ins provide an opportunity to recalibrate your plans, ensuring that they remain aligned with your long-term objectives and current needs. By engaging in this practice, you'll develop a deeper understanding of your work habits and how to optimize them.

Interactive Element: Weekly Planner Reflection

At the end of each week, take a few minutes to review your planner. Reflect on what went well and where you encountered challenges. Consider the following questions: What tasks did I complete, and what did I learn from them? Were there any distractions that could be minimized in the future? How did I feel about my workload and its balance with personal time? Use your insights to make adjustments for the coming week, refining your approach and continually improving your time management skills. This reflection not only enhances productivity but also fosters a sense of accomplishment and growth.

DIGITAL TOOLS FOR TIME MANAGEMENT

Navigating the digital landscape can feel like wandering through a bustling city without a map, especially when ADHD makes focusing on tasks a bit like trying to catch a lightning bug in a jar. However, digital tools have become the modern-day compass, guiding us through the maze of deadlines, appointments, and endless to-do lists. Task management apps are at the forefront of this revolution, offering a structured yet flexible way to organize our daily chaos. Apps like Todoist, Asana, and Trello provide platforms where you can create tasks, set priorities, and track progress with a finger swipe. They cater to the ADHD brain by breaking down overwhelming projects into bite-sized pieces, making them seem less daunting. Calendar integrations further enhance this setup by syncing schedules across devices, ensuring that reminders pop up exactly when needed, whether you're at your desk or on the go. This seamless coordination between task managers and calendars can be a game-changer, helping to bridge the gap between planning and execution.

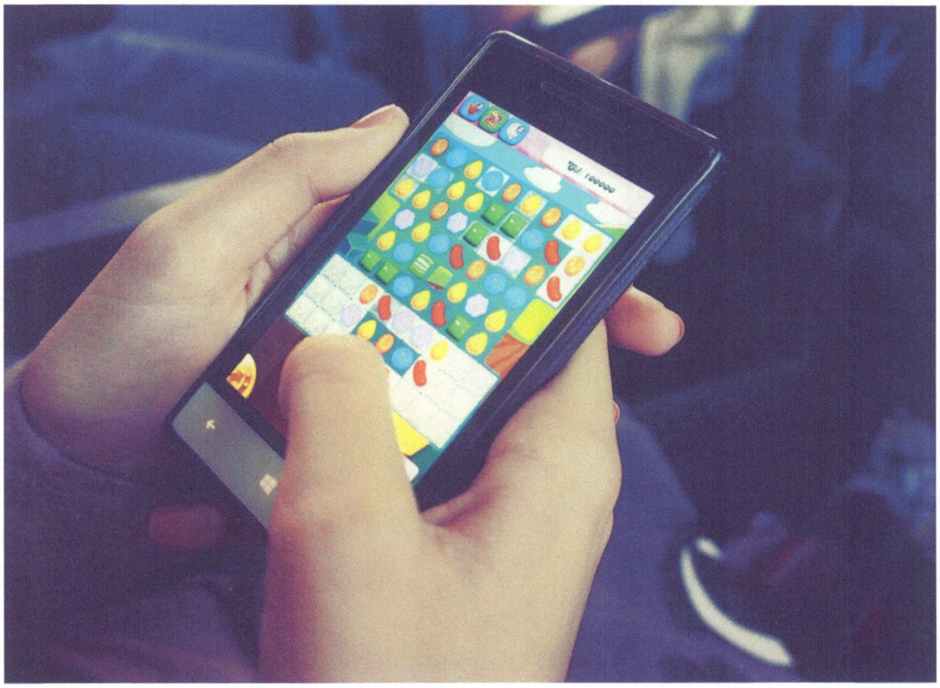

Choosing the right digital tools is a bit like finding the perfect pair of shoes—what works for one person might not work for another. It's important to consider what features are most crucial for your needs. Simplicity in the user interface is key, especially for those of us who may get distracted by too many options or a cluttered screen. Look for apps that offer a clean layout along with straightforward navigation. Customization options are another vital feature, allowing you to tailor alerts and reminders to your specific preferences. Maybe you need a gentle nudge every hour to refocus, or perhaps a bold reminder each morning to prioritize your tasks for the day. The ability to adjust these settings means the tool can work with your unique rhythms and requirements—rather than against them.

Once you've selected your digital toolkit, the next step is to weave these tools into the fabric of your daily life. Consistency is crucial here, and syncing across devices ensures that you have access to your schedule and tasks no matter where you are. This kind of integration supports a cohesive approach to time management, eliminating the need to juggle multiple platforms or remember where you noted down that important deadline. Setting up daily reminders can also help keep you on track. Whether it's an alert to start your morning routine or a ping reminding you to take a break, these little prompts act as checkpoints throughout your day, guiding you back to your priorities when distractions threaten to pull you off course.

As with any tool, evaluating effectiveness is a critical step in ensuring that you're getting the most out of your digital aids. Regular feedback loops are an excellent way to assess how well these tools are serving you. Take a moment at the end of each week to review your productivity metrics. Did you complete more tasks than the previous week? Were there fewer days when you felt overwhelmed by your schedule? Comparing these metrics before and after implementing digital tools can provide valuable insights into their impact. If something isn't working as expected, don't hesitate to make adjustments. Maybe a different app would suit your style better, or perhaps tweaking your reminder settings could boost your productivity. This process of evaluation and adjustment is ongoing, reflecting the dynamic nature of ADHD and the need for flexible solutions.

Digital tools are not a one-size-fits-all solution, but they can be powerful, supportive allies in the quest to tame time management challenges. By exploring the available options, selecting those that align with your personal needs, and integrating them into your daily life, you can create a robust framework that supports your unique way of working. As you fine-tune this system, you'll likely find that managing your time becomes less about struggling to keep up—and more about confidently steering your course.

OVERCOMING PROCRASTINATION WITH THE TWO-MINUTE RULE

Procrastination is a familiar nemesis for many of us with ADHD, often lurking in the shadows of our to-do lists, ready to pounce when we least expect it. It's not just a matter of being lazy or careless; it's a complex dance between task aversion and decision paralysis. Task aversion creeps in when a task seems too daunting or boring, making it hard to even start. Our brains seek out more rewarding activities, leaving the dreaded tasks to pile up like a mountain we can't climb. Decision paralysis adds to this by trapping us in a cycle of indecision, where even choosing what to tackle first becomes an insurmountable challenge. This paralysis can turn a simple decision into an all-consuming dilemma, leaving us feeling stuck and overwhelmed.

Enter the Two-Minute Rule, a straightforward yet powerful technique that offers a lifeline out of the procrastination quicksand. The premise is simple: if a task takes two minutes or less to complete, do it immediately. This strategy works wonders for those quick wins—like replying to an email, tidying up your desk, or jotting down a meeting note. But its power extends beyond just small tasks. The Two-Minute Rule can also serve as a gateway, helping you break into larger projects. By committing to just two minutes on a bigger task, you often find that once you've started, the momentum carries you forward, and what seemed insurmountable becomes manageable. This approach helps bypass the initial resistance and gets the ball rolling, turning potential procrastination into productive action.

The beauty of this technique lies in its ability to build momentum, creating a ripple effect that propels you through your day. Each small task completed is a win—a boost of motivation that encourages you to keep going. As these small victories accumulate, they chip away at the overwhelming mountain of tasks, reducing it to a series of manageable steps. This continuous sense of achievement can be incredibly motivating, making it easier to transition to more complex tasks. The Two-Minute Rule acts as a catalyst, sparking the initial action needed to dive into larger projects without feeling paralyzed by their scope. It's about finding that first crack in the wall of procrastination and using it to widen the gap until the wall crumbles altogether.

The long-term benefits of consistently applying the Two-Minute Rule are significant. By incorporating this concept into your daily routine, you may notice a marked increase in task initiation, making it easier to start and finish tasks without hesitation. This improvement can lead to a substantial reduction in your task backlog, as those pesky two-minute tasks no longer linger on your to-do list, haunting you day after day. Over time, this can lead to a more organized and less cluttered life, freeing up mental space for creativity and growth. The cumulative effect is a more proactive approach to managing your responsibilities, where procrastination loses its power and productivity becomes your default setting.

As we wrap up this chapter, let's take a moment to reflect on the tools we've explored for mastering time management. From structuring your day with the Pomodoro Technique to harnessing the focus of visual planners and digital tools, each strategy offers a unique way to navigate the complexities of ADHD. They provide a framework that supports productivity while allowing for flexibility and personalization. As you integrate these techniques into your life, you'll find that managing time becomes less about battling against the clock and more about working with the rhythms of your ADHD mind.

This sets the stage for our next exploration, where we'll dive into the realm of emotional regulation—a key piece in the puzzle of living well with ADHD.

CHAPTER 3
ENHANCING EMOTIONAL REGULATION

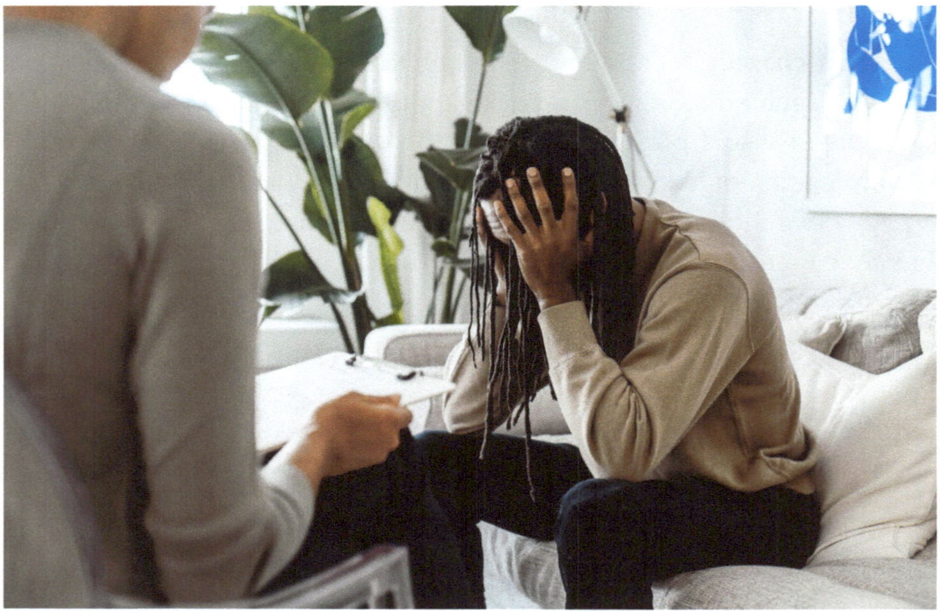

EMOTIONAL REGULATION with ADHD often feels like riding a rollercoaster blindfolded—never quite knowing when the next twist or drop will hit. I used to find myself in the middle of conversations, feeling the heat rise in my cheeks as a wave of frustration or anxiety washed over me. It was as if my emotions had a mind of their own, hijacking my thoughts and leaving me scrambling to regain control. This unpredictable emotional landscape is something many of us with ADHD know all too well, and it can be exhausting. But there's a tool that has helped me—and countless others—find a sense of calm amidst the chaos: mindfulness.

Mindfulness is gaining attention as a powerful tool for those of us with ADHD. It's a practice rooted in present-moment awareness, asking us to tune into what's happening right now, without letting our minds wander to the past or future. For individuals with ADHD—whose thoughts often feel like a never-ending game of pinball—mindfulness offers a reprieve. It helps you focus and relax, providing a mental anchor when you're feeling adrift. Science supports the benefits of mindfulness, with studies indicating it can induce changes in brain areas linked to attention and emotion regulation. By practicing mindfulness, you can reduce activity in the brain's default mode network, which is responsible for mind-wandering and often in overdrive in ADHD brains. This makes mindfulness not just a calming practice but a way to strengthen your mental faculties.

Incorporating mindfulness strategies into your daily routine doesn't require grand gestures or hours of meditation. It can be as simple as taking a few moments each day to practice mindful breathing. When you find yourself feeling overwhelmed, pause and take a deep breath. Focus on each inhale and exhale, letting your mind settle on the rhythm of your breath. This practice can bring immediate calm, like a reset button for your brain.

Another effective exercise is the body scan meditation, where you mentally check the status of each part of your body, noticing any tension and gently releasing it. This not only enhances awareness but also helps you connect with your physical self, grounding you in the present moment. Even a walk can become a mindful experience. As you stroll, engage your senses by noticing the colors of the leaves, the sound of your footsteps, or the feel of the breeze on your skin. Mindful walking transforms a mundane activity into a sensory exploration, drawing your focus back to the here and now.

Creating mindful moments throughout the day can help you maintain that sense of calm and focus, even amidst life's demands. One way to do this is by setting reminders for mindfulness breaks. These can be simple prompts on your phone or sticky notes placed around your workspace, gently nudging you to pause and breathe. Mindfulness apps can also be invaluable, offering guided sessions that fit into any schedule. They provide structure and support, making it easier to commit to regular practice. By intentionally carving out time for mindfulness, you create a buffer against stress and emotional upheaval, building resilience one moment at a time.

The benefits of regular mindfulness practice extend far beyond immediate calm. Over time, mindfulness can lead to reduced stress and anxiety, providing a stable foundation for daily life. Improved concentration is another significant benefit, as mindfulness strengthens your ability to focus on tasks without getting sidetracked. Emotional stability also improves, helping you respond to situations with greater composure and less reactivity. For those of us with ADHD, who often feel at the mercy of our emotions, this stability is a game-changer. It's like finding a steady handhold on a rocky path, giving you the confidence to navigate life's challenges with ease.

Interactive Element: Mindfulness Practice Checklist

To help you get started, here's a simple checklist of mindfulness practices you can incorporate into your routine. Choose one or two to try each day:

- Mindful Breathing: Take five deep breaths, focusing on the sensation of each inhale and exhale.
- Body Scan Meditation: Spend five minutes mentally scanning your body from head to toe, noticing areas of tension and releasing them.
- Mindful Walking: On your next walk, engage your senses by observing sights, sounds, and physical sensations.
- Mindfulness Breaks: Set reminders to pause and breathe for a minute every hour.
- Use a Mindful App: Download an app like Headspace or Calm and explore their guided sessions.

By making mindfulness a regular part of your life, you'll find that it becomes a trusted companion, always there to help you center yourself whenever you need it. Personally, I recommend that clients with ADHD do 10 minutes of meditation a day to help with emotional regulation and focus. I do 20 minutes a day, and I've noticed a difference in my mood and my ability to organize my day and week schedule.

EMOTIONAL AWARENESS: IDENTIFYING TRIGGERS

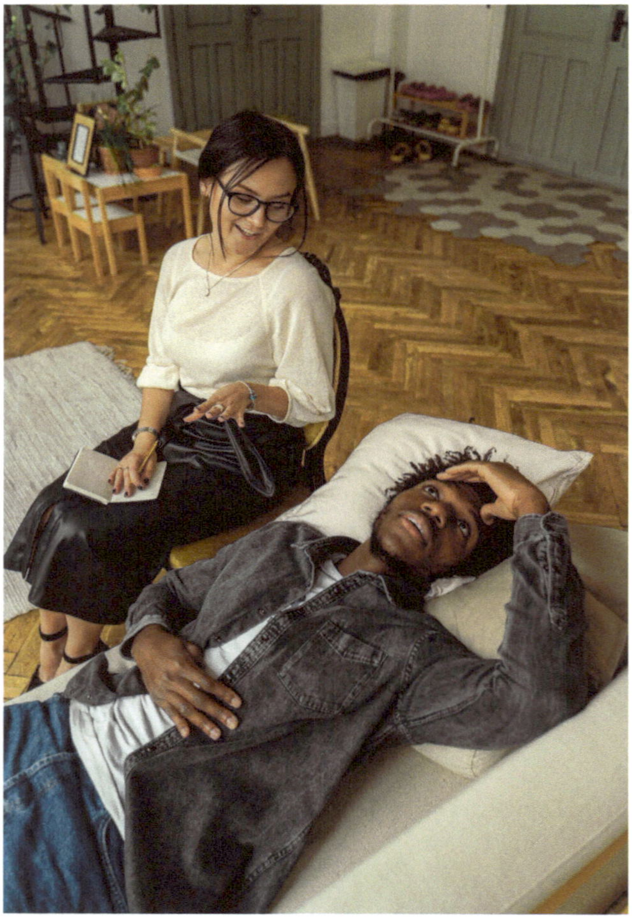

Emotional triggers can feel like hidden landmines scattered through our daily lives, waiting to erupt with little warning. They are the raw nerves that, when touched, unleash a cascade of emotional responses that can catch even the most prepared among us off guard. These triggers are often rooted in both physiological and psychological origins. Physiologically, our bodies react to certain stimuli—think of the adrenaline spike when startled or the knot in your stomach during stress. Psychologically, past experiences play a critical role in forming these triggers. Memories of past events, especially those tied to intense emotions like fear or anger, can imprint on our psyche, creating patterns that influence how we react to similar situations in the present. Recognizing how these elements interplay can provide valuable insight into our emotional responses.

Identifying your personal triggers is a crucial step in managing them. It's like assembling a map of your emotional landscape, one that highlights the terrain you must navigate. Keeping an emotional journal can be an enlightening practice. Write down moments when you feel a strong emotional response, noting what happened, how you felt, and any physical sensations that accompanied it. Over time, patterns will emerge, revealing specific scenarios or interactions that consistently provoke a reaction. Reflecting on these entries helps you pinpoint the triggers you might not have been consciously aware of. Additionally, consider how your body responds—perhaps your heart races, your muscles tense, or you feel a flush of heat. These physiological cues are signals that your amygdala, the brain's emotional center, is activated, preparing for a fight, flight, or freeze response.

Once you've identified your triggers, managing your reactions becomes a more achievable task. One of the simplest yet most effective strategies is to incorporate breathing techniques. When you sense a trigger approaching, take a deep breath, hold it for a moment, and then release it slowly. This simple act can activate your parasympathetic nervous system, helping to calm your body and mind. Developing a trigger response plan can also be beneficial. This plan might include steps like removing yourself from the situation, redirecting your focus, or using grounding techniques to bring your attention back to the present. Engaging in constructive self-talk is another powerful tool. In moments of heightened emotion, remind yourself that it's okay to feel what you're feeling and that you have the tools to manage it. Phrases like "This too shall pass" or "I can handle this" can provide reassurance and prevent you from being swept away by the emotional tide.

Developing emotional awareness is like sharpening a tool that allows you to navigate your emotional world with greater precision. It involves recognizing the early signs of emotional upheaval before they escalate. This could mean noticing a slight increase in your heart rate or a change in your thought patterns. By catching these signs early, you give yourself the opportunity to intervene before the situation spirals. Practicing emotional labeling is a technique that can bring clarity to your emotional state. By naming the emotions you're experiencing—whether it's frustration, sadness, or excitement—you can create a sense of distance from them. This distance allows you to observe your emotions without being consumed by them, fostering a sense of control and understanding.

Interactive Element: Emotional Trigger Journal

To enhance your emotional awareness, consider starting a journal dedicated to tracking your emotional triggers. Begin by noting down each incident where you experienced a strong emotional reaction. Include details such as the situation, your thoughts and feelings, physical sensations, and any actions you took. Reflect on these entries regularly, looking for patterns in your triggers and responses. This practice not only helps you identify your personal triggers but also enables you to develop a proactive approach to managing them. By understanding your emotional landscape, you gain the power to navigate it with confidence and resilience.

SELF-COMPASSION: THE ART OF BEING KIND TO YOURSELF

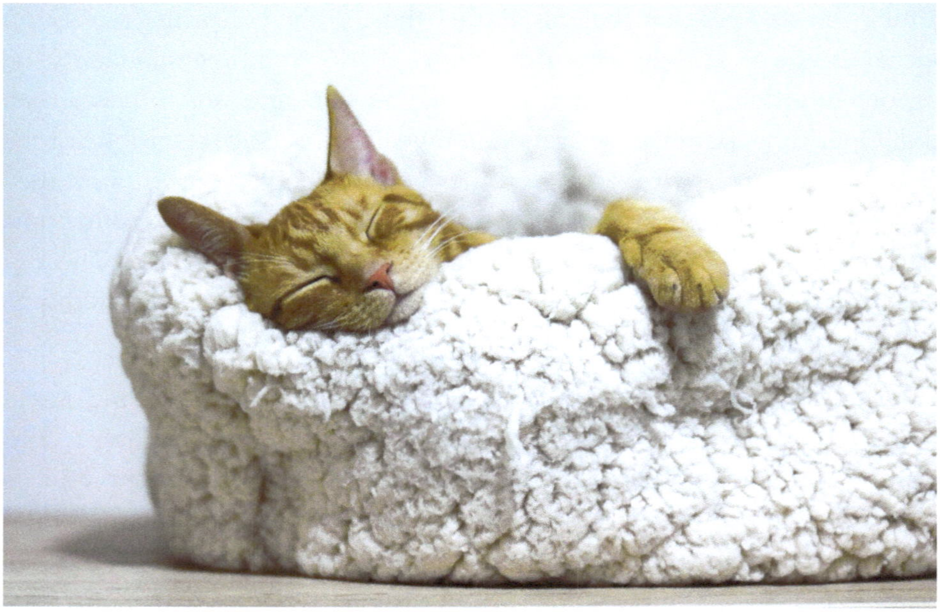

Living with ADHD can sometimes feel like being in a **perpetual tug-of-war** with your own mind. There are days when you might feel like you're not measuring up to your own expectations—or those of others. In these moments, **self-compassion** is more than just a comforting notion; it's a **lifeline**. The relentless self-criticism that often accompanies ADHD can erode your confidence and self-worth, leading you to internalize stigmas that paint ADHD as a flaw rather than a different way of thinking. When you practice self-compassion, you open the door to reducing this harsh self-judgment, allowing yourself to see your struggles through a **kinder lens**. It's about acknowledging that everyone faces challenges and that having ADHD doesn't define your value. This shift in perspective is vital to building a **positive self-image**, where you recognize your strengths alongside your weaknesses.

Integrating self-compassion into daily life can start with simple exercises that gradually reshape how you view yourself. One powerful practice is **writing a letter to yourself**. Imagine you're speaking to a dear friend who's feeling down, and extend that same kindness and understanding to yourself. Write about your struggles and achievements, expressing empathy and encouragement. This exercise can be profoundly healing, offering a moment of **reflection and self-acceptance**.

Daily affirmations also play a crucial role in nurturing self-kindness. Affirmations are positive statements that you repeat to yourself, reinforcing a compassionate and supportive mindset. Phrases like *"I am worthy of love and respect"* or *"I am doing my best, and that's enough"* can ground you in self-acceptance, especially when negative thoughts threaten to take hold.

Another aspect of self-compassion is **setting realistic goals** that acknowledge your unique pace and abilities. By aligning your goals with what's genuinely achievable, you reduce the pressure to conform to unrealistic standards, making room for **growth and joy** in the process.

Overcoming self-judgment is a journey of **unlearning the harsh narratives** you may have internalized. It involves actively reframing negative thoughts and challenging the assumptions that fuel them. When you catch yourself thinking, *"I'm such a failure for missing that deadline,"* pause and reframe it to, *"I faced a challenge, and I can learn from this experience."* This shift from **self-criticism to constructive reflection** can transform setbacks into opportunities for growth.

Understanding **perfectionism and its pitfalls** is another crucial step. Perfectionism often masquerades as a motivator, but in reality, it sets unattainable standards that can lead to exhaustion and self-doubt. By recognizing that **perfection isn't the goal**, you free yourself to embrace imperfections and celebrate progress—no matter how small. This mindset shift fosters **resilience**, allowing you to bounce back from mistakes with a renewed sense of purpose and determination.

The **long-term benefits** of practicing self-compassion extend beyond immediate relief from self-criticism. Over time, self-compassion can enhance your **emotional resilience**, equipping you to face life's challenges with greater ease and adaptability. When you treat yourself with kindness, you build a foundation of **inner strength** that supports you through ups and downs. This resilience doesn't mean you won't encounter difficulties, but it does mean you'll be better prepared to navigate them without losing your sense of self-worth.

Additionally, self-compassion contributes to greater **life satisfaction and contentment**. By accepting yourself fully—flaws and all—you cultivate a sense of **peace and fulfillment** that isn't dependent on external validation. This internal harmony allows you to engage more authentically with the world, fostering **deeper connections** and a **richer experience of life**.

Interactive Element: Self-Compassion Letter Exercise

Take a moment to write a letter to yourself. Begin by acknowledging any challenges you're currently facing, and then offer words of kindness and understanding as you would to a friend. Reflect on your strengths and the progress you've made, no matter how small. Encourage yourself to keep moving forward with compassion and patience. Revisit this letter whenever you need a reminder of your worth and resilience. This exercise is a step towards embracing self-compassion as a daily practice, nurturing a positive self-image, and a kinder relationship with yourself.

BUILDING RESILIENCE: BOUNCING BACK STRONGER

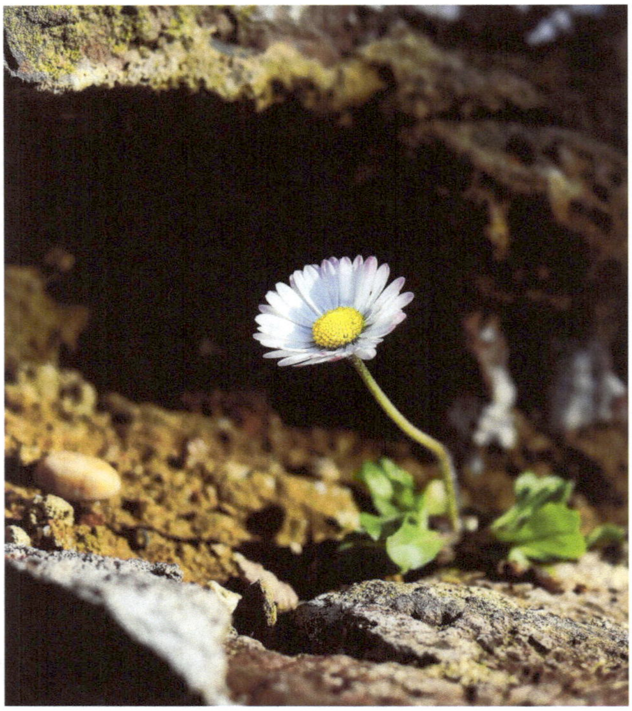

Resilience is like that invisible muscle we all have, allowing us to bounce back when life throws us a curveball. For those of us managing ADHD, resilience plays a crucial role in maintaining our mental health. Think of it as the ability to recover from setbacks and adapt to difficult situations. It's not about never failing, but rather about how we respond when things don't go as planned. When you cultivate resilience, you're better equipped to manage stress, overcome obstacles, and maintain a sense of control—even when everything feels overwhelming. This ability to recover and adapt is foundational for emotional regulation, helping you navigate the highs and lows more smoothly.

Building resilience involves setting and achieving small, incremental goals. These goals act as stepping stones, helping you move forward without feeling overwhelmed. Start with something simple, like organizing a small part of your home or completing a single work task. Each accomplished goal boosts your confidence and reinforces your ability to tackle more significant challenges. By focusing on these smaller victories, you gradually build a pattern of success and resilience.

Additionally, cultivating a support network is vital. Surround yourself with people who understand your challenges and can offer encouragement and perspective. Whether it's family, friends, or a support group, having a network provides a safety net when times get tough, allowing you to share burdens and celebrate achievements.

Engaging in problem-solving exercises can significantly enhance your resilience. Problem-solving encourages you to approach challenges methodically, breaking them down into manageable parts. This might involve brainstorming solutions, weighing the pros and cons, or seeking advice from others. By practicing problem-solving regularly, you train your brain to handle adversity with creativity and confidence. It's about developing a toolkit of strategies that you can rely on when faced with difficulties, making you more adaptable and less likely to be derailed by unexpected events. These exercises are like regular workouts for your resilience muscle, strengthening it over time.

Real-life stories of resilience can be incredibly inspiring, especially for those of us navigating ADHD. Consider someone who, despite struggling with organization and deadlines, has built a successful career. They may have faced numerous setbacks, yet each one taught them valuable lessons about time management and prioritization. Overcoming these challenges required persistence and adaptability, qualities that are at the heart of resilience. Another example might involve someone who, after years of battling self-doubt, learned to channel their unique strengths into creative pursuits, finding fulfillment and success. These stories remind us that resilience is not just about survival—but about using adversity as a catalyst for growth and transformation.

Fostering a growth mindset is a powerful way to build resilience. This mindset encourages you to see challenges as opportunities for development rather than insurmountable obstacles. Embracing failures as learning experiences allows you to grow from every setback, transforming potential roadblocks into stepping stones. By focusing on progress rather than perfection, you cultivate a sense of resilience that propels you forward. Celebrate each step forward—no matter how small—and acknowledge the effort you've put into your journey. This approach not only builds resilience but also enhances your overall well-being, fostering a sense of satisfaction and accomplishment in your daily life.

So, as we wrap up this chapter on emotional regulation, remember that resilience is your ally. It's the strength that helps you weather life's storms and come out even stronger. By setting achievable goals, building a supportive network, and embracing a growth mindset, you're equipping yourself with the tools to navigate any challenge. With resilience, you're not just bouncing back—you're bouncing forward, ready to tackle whatever comes next.

In the following chapter, we'll explore how nurturing relationships can further enhance your journey, providing stability and support.

CHAPTER 4
NURTURING RELATIONSHIPS

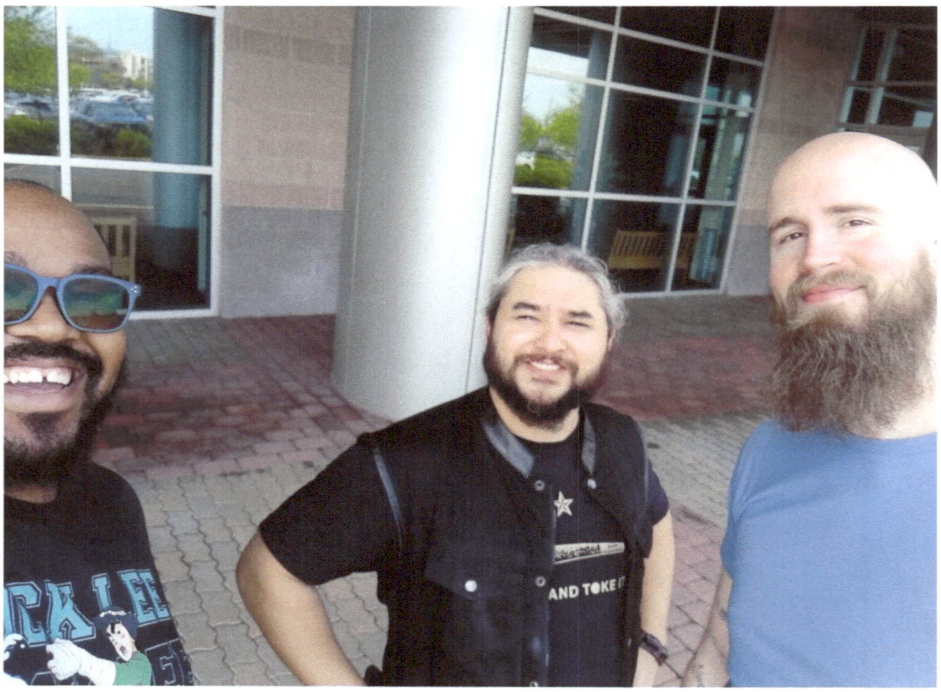

Ocean City Comic-Con 2023 - left to right (Myself, Jesús "Jesse" Cruz, Samuel "Sam" Cain) we have regular virtual guys night to chat and play video games.

I REMEMBER the first time I realized communication wasn't just about talking. I was in a heated discussion with a colleague, and despite all my logical points, the conversation felt like two ships passing in the night. My thoughts were clear in my head but somehow tangled on their way out. That's when it hit me—communication is as much about listening and understanding as it is about expressing. For those of us with ADHD, this realization can be a game changer. Effective communication isn't just about getting your point across; it's about connection, empathy, and clarity.

At the heart of clear and empathetic communication is active listening. This isn't just hearing words; it's about truly understanding what the other person is saying. It's about being present and giving the speaker your full attention, something that can be challenging with ADHD when distractions lurk everywhere. Start by maintaining eye contact, which can help anchor your focus. Nod occasionally to show you're engaged. Repeat back what you've heard to confirm understanding, saying things like, "So what you're saying is..." or "I hear you feel...". This reflective listening technique assures the speaker that you're with them, not just waiting for your turn to speak. Non-verbal cues also play a significant role. Your body language, facial expressions, and even the tone of your voice all convey messages that words alone can't capture. A warm smile or a concerned nod can speak volumes, bridging gaps that words can't cross.

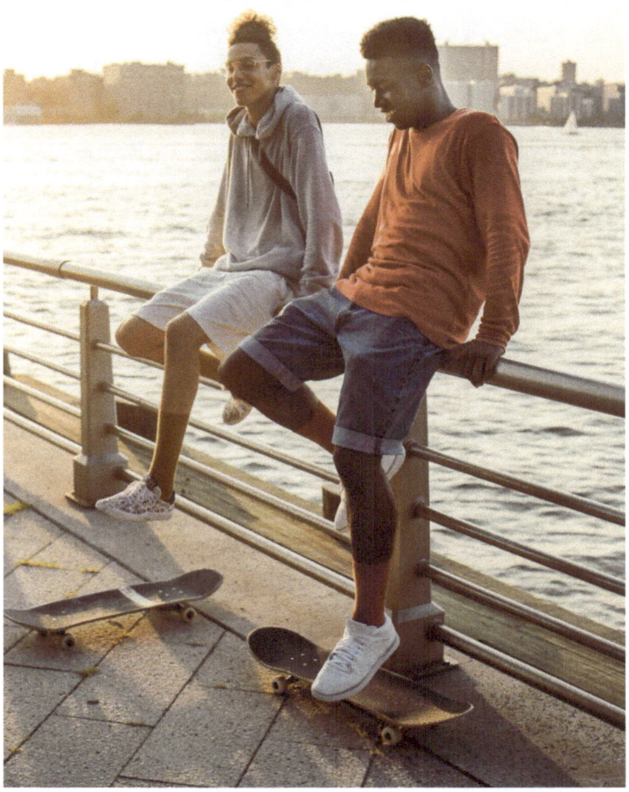

When it comes time to express your own thoughts and feelings, clarity is key. This means using "I" statements to articulate your needs and emotions. Instead of saying, "You never listen to me," try, "I feel unheard when you interrupt me." This subtle shift focuses on your feelings rather than assigning blame, reducing defensiveness and opening the door to more productive dialogue. Simplifying your language can also prevent misunderstandings. Be clear and concise, avoiding jargon or complex explanations that can muddy the waters. When your message is straightforward, it's more likely to be understood as intended, minimizing confusion and misinterpretation.

Practicing empathy in conversations transforms ordinary exchanges into meaningful connections. Empathy isn't about agreeing with someone; it's about understanding their perspective. Engage in reflective listening exercises, where you intentionally put yourself in the other person's shoes. Ask open-ended questions to encourage them to elaborate on their feelings and thoughts. Empathy mapping can also be a valuable tool. This involves considering what the other person might be thinking, feeling, and experiencing, allowing you to connect with their emotions more deeply. By fostering this level of understanding, you build trust and rapport, laying the foundation for stronger, more resilient relationships.

ADHD presents unique communication challenges that can sometimes feel like an uphill battle. Conversation drift is a common hurdle, where your mind wanders mid-discussion, leaving your conversational partner bewildered. To combat this, practice grounding techniques like focusing on a specific word or phrase to bring your attention back. If you feel yourself veering off-topic, gently steer the conversation back by acknowledging the drift and redirecting focus. Strategies for staying on topic can also include setting clear objectives for the conversation. Before diving in, outline the key points you want to cover, keeping them visible as a reference. This can help anchor the discussion and keep you aligned with your goals.

Interactive Element: Communication Self-Assessment

Consider taking a moment to reflect on your own communication style. Think about a recent conversation—did you actively listen, or were you more focused on what you wanted to say next? How clear were you in expressing your thoughts and feelings? Did you practice empathy, seeking to understand the other person's perspective? By evaluating your strengths and areas for improvement, you can develop a more effective communication style that fosters connection and understanding. This awareness is the first step toward nurturing relationships that thrive on clarity and empathy.

Effective communication is not just a skill; it's a bridge that connects us to others. By honing these techniques, you can transform conversations into opportunities for deeper connection and understanding. In the following sections, we'll continue to explore how nurturing relationships can enhance your life, providing stability and support in deeply resonated ways.

MANAGING MISUNDERSTANDINGS AND CONFLICTS

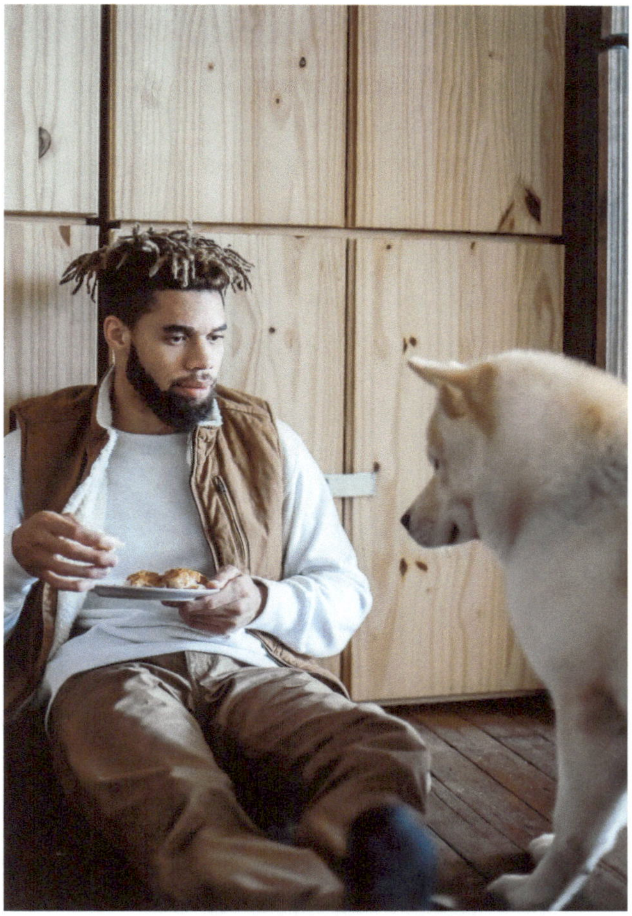

Misunderstandings in relationships, particularly those involving ADHD, can often feel like shadowy figures lurking just beyond the light of clear communication. They tend to arise from misinterpretations of intentions, where words and actions are misconstrued, resulting in hurt feelings and confusion. Imagine a scenario where you forget an important date or misplace a significant item. To someone without ADHD, these might seem like careless oversights, but for you, they could be the result of a chaotic mental landscape. This difference in perception can lead to accusations of neglect or indifference when, in reality, your intentions were quite the opposite.

Stress-induced miscommunication adds another layer of complexity. When stress levels rise, communication can become fraught with tension, leading to defensive reactions and impulsive comments. In such moments, the true message often gets lost in the emotional turmoil, leaving both parties feeling misunderstood and alienated.

Resolving conflicts constructively requires a toolbox of techniques tailored to navigate these choppy waters. Compromise plays a crucial role, acting as the bridge between differing perspectives. It involves meeting halfway, acknowledging that both parties have valid points, and recognizing that a solution can often be found in the middle ground. It's about letting go of the need to be right and focusing on finding a mutually satisfying resolution.

Sometimes, when tempers flare and emotions run high, a time-out strategy can be invaluable. Taking a break allows everyone to cool down and gain perspective before returning to the discussion with a calmer mindset. This pause can prevent the situation from escalating and give space for reflection.

Mediation practices with a neutral third party can also be beneficial, particularly when the conflict feels insurmountable. A mediator can offer an unbiased perspective, facilitating open dialogue and guiding the conversation toward resolution.

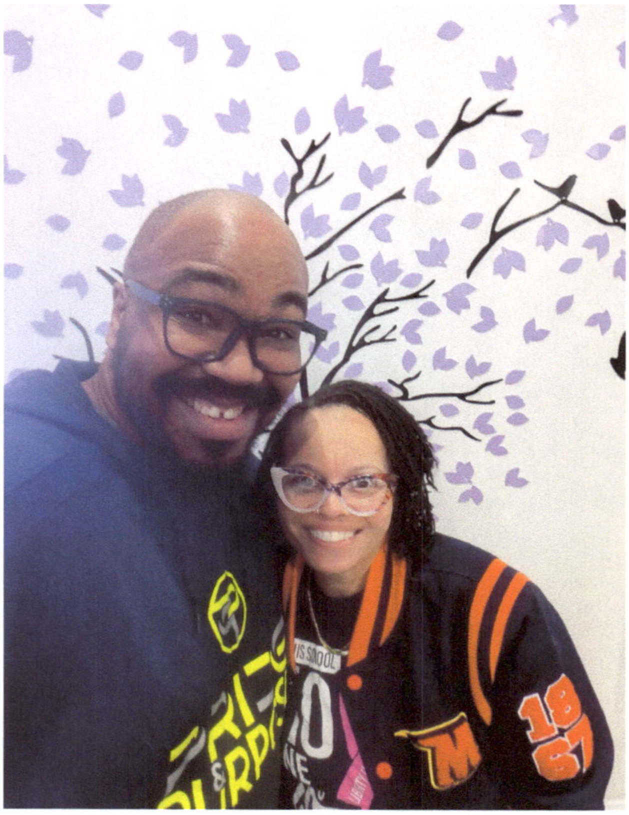

(Myself and my mentor Terri E. Johnson "TJ" Author of *Body Safety Zones (BSZ)* @persistenceistheway)

Repairing relationship strains after a conflict is akin to rebuilding a bridge that has been partially washed away. It requires patience, effort, and the willingness to mend what was damaged. An apology framework can provide a solid foundation for genuine reconciliation. A meaningful apology goes beyond a simple "I'm sorry." It involves expressing remorse, acknowledging the impact of your actions, and offering a plan for change. This approach demonstrates accountability and a commitment to healing the relationship.

Building trust through consistent actions is another vital component. Trust is fragile and can be easily broken, but it can be rebuilt through repeated, reliable behavior. Keeping promises, being dependable, and showing respect for the other person's feelings all contribute to restoring trust over time. It's about proving through actions, not just words, that the relationship is valued and worth nurturing.

Preventing future conflicts is an ongoing process that involves laying a groundwork of clear communication expectations. This means discussing and agreeing on how you will communicate—especially during disagreements. Will you set aside time for regular check-ins to address concerns before they escalate? These check-ins can act as safety valves, releasing pressure and preventing small issues from snowballing into full-blown conflicts.

By establishing a routine for open conversations, you create a space where both parties can express their needs and frustrations without fear of judgment. This proactive approach fosters a sense of security and understanding, reducing the likelihood of misunderstandings and conflicts down the line. It's like maintaining a garden—regular attention and care can prevent weeds from taking over, allowing the relationship to flourish.

ADHD AND INTIMACY: STRENGTHENING BONDS

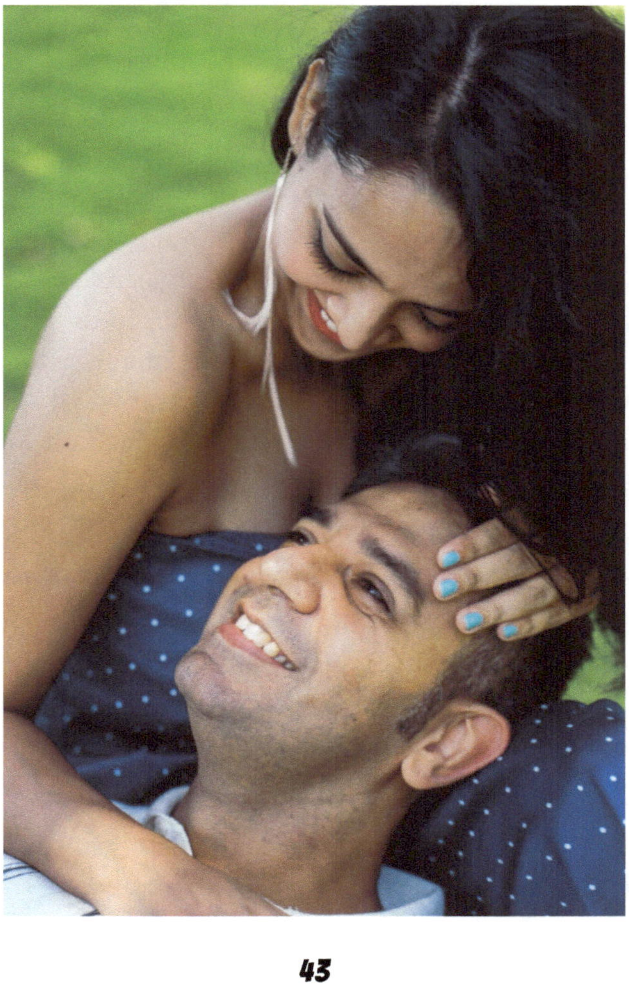

ADHD in intimate relationships can feel like both a blessing and a challenge. The spontaneity and creativity that often come with ADHD can invigorate a relationship, adding excitement and unpredictability. However, these traits can also introduce complexities, particularly when it comes to sensory sensitivities and emotional connection. Sensory sensitivities might mean that certain textures, sounds, or lights become overwhelming, affecting comfort levels during intimate moments. Perhaps the hum of a ceiling fan becomes a relentless distraction, or the feel of certain fabrics against the skin is irritating. These seemingly small details can disrupt the peace and focus required for intimacy, leading to frustration on both sides.

Emotional intimacy also presents challenges, as ADHD can sometimes make it difficult to express emotions clearly or consistently. There might be times when thoughts and feelings feel tangled, making it hard to open up or connect deeply with a partner. This can create a sense of distance, even when the love is strong, leaving both partners searching for a bridge across the gap.

Deepening emotional connections requires intentional effort and understanding. One effective strategy is to schedule quality time together. This doesn't have to be elaborate; it could be as simple as a regular evening walk or a weekly coffee date. The key is consistency, creating a space where you and your partner can connect without distractions. During these times, share stories and experiences that matter to you. Talk about your day, your dreams, your fears. This sharing builds a foundation of trust and understanding, where both partners feel seen and valued. It's about carving out moments where you can truly be present with each other, away from the noise of the outside world. These shared experiences become the threads that weave a more profound emotional tapestry, strengthening the bond between you.

Intimacy challenges, especially managing distractions during intimate moments, are common—but not insurmountable. ADHD often means that your mind is a bustling place, full of thoughts and ideas jostling for attention. In intimate settings, this can lead to a drift in focus, which might make your partner feel neglected or disconnected. Mindfulness can be a powerful tool to counter this. By practicing mindfulness, you train your attention to remain in the moment, allowing you to fully engage with your partner. This might involve simple breathing exercises to center yourself or focusing on the sensations of touch and sound to ground your attention. Mindfulness helps create an intimate space where distractions fade and presence takes center stage. It's about being there—truly there—with your partner, embracing the moment together.

Building a stronger partnership involves more than just managing challenges; it's about actively fostering a supportive and collaborative relationship. One way to do this is through collaborative goal setting. Sit down with your partner and discuss your shared goals, both big and small. Whether it's planning a vacation, deciding on savings targets, or even dividing household responsibilities, working together to set and achieve goals strengthens your partnership. It creates a sense of teamwork, where both partners feel equally invested and responsible.

Celebrating milestones is also crucial. Recognize and celebrate the achievements you reach together, whether they're personal accomplishments or shared goals. This could be as simple as acknowledging your partner's hard work with a heartfelt note or planning a special dinner to mark a significant moment. Celebrations are not just about the big wins, but also about appreciating the journey you've taken together.

Intimacy, in all its forms, thrives on understanding, presence, and shared experiences. By addressing the challenges that ADHD might introduce and focusing on enhancing emotional bonds, you can create a relationship that is not only resilient but also deeply fulfilling. It's about seeing each other fully and choosing to connect day after day, even when the path isn't always smooth.

BUILDING A SUPPORTIVE COMMUNITY

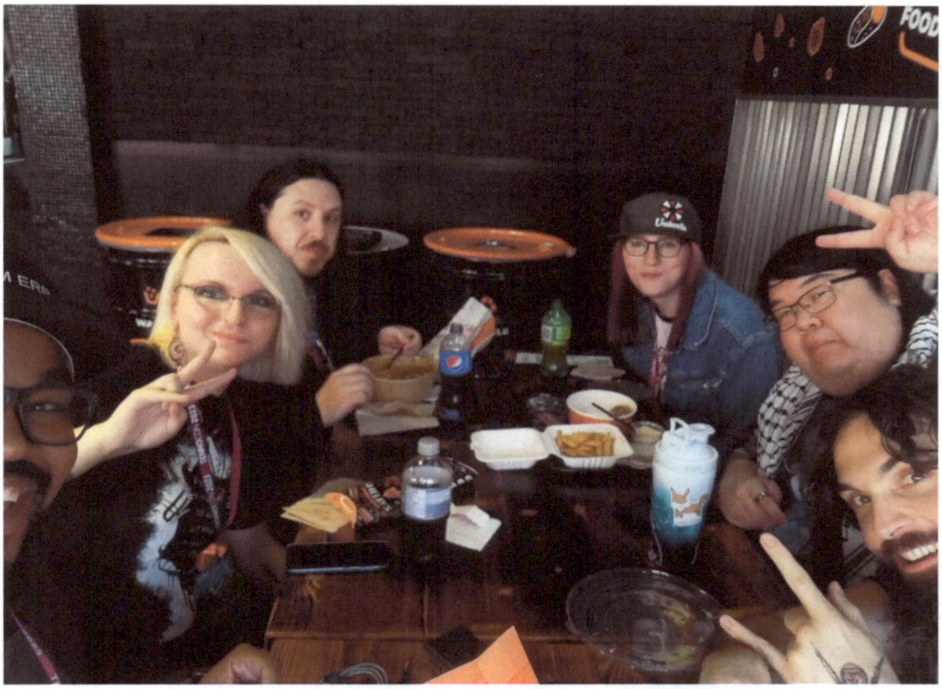

Left to right (Myself, Voice Quills, Stoic_Nod, Miabyte, Pixel Panda, Antonio Greco aka the voice of "Erra" at Tennocon 2023 for the game Warframe)

Living with ADHD often feels like navigating a maze with ever-changing walls, and having a supportive community is like having a group of friends with flashlights helping you find your way. Community support provides emotional reassurance and understanding in a world that sometimes feels unsympathetic to the nuances of ADHD. It's about connecting with people who genuinely get it and who know that a chaotic mind doesn't equate to a lack of care or effort. This mutual understanding is incredibly comforting, offering a safe space where you don't have to explain or justify your experiences. In these communities, shared resources and experiences form the backbone of support. Whether it's exchanging tips on managing impulsivity or sharing a laugh over common ADHD quirks, these interactions light the path forward and remind you that you're not alone in your challenges.

Finding your tribe and those who resonate with your experiences can be a transformative step. Start by exploring local support groups or meetups where you can physically connect with others facing similar challenges. These gatherings provide an opportunity to share stories and strategies in a setting that's designed for empathy and support. If in-person meetings aren't feasible, online forums and social media communities can serve as a virtual haven. Platforms like Reddit or Facebook host numerous ADHD groups, offering a space to ask questions, exchange advice, and build friendships with people worldwide. Networking at ADHD conferences and workshops is another way to deepen your connections. These events bring together experts, advocates, and individuals living with ADHD, creating a vibrant environment ripe for learning and interaction. It's about finding those who speak your language and can share in your victories and setbacks.

Contributing to your community by getting involved can be incredibly rewarding, both for you and those you support. Volunteering at community events or within support groups not only helps others but also strengthens your ties to the community. Sharing personal insights and experiences can inspire and guide others on their ADHD path. Perhaps you've developed a unique strategy for managing time or found a mindfulness practice that calms your mind. Passing on these insights can make a big difference for someone else. Your experiences, both struggles and successes, add to the collective wisdom of the group, creating a rich tapestry of shared knowledge. This proactive involvement fosters a sense of belonging and purpose, showing that everyone has something valuable to contribute.

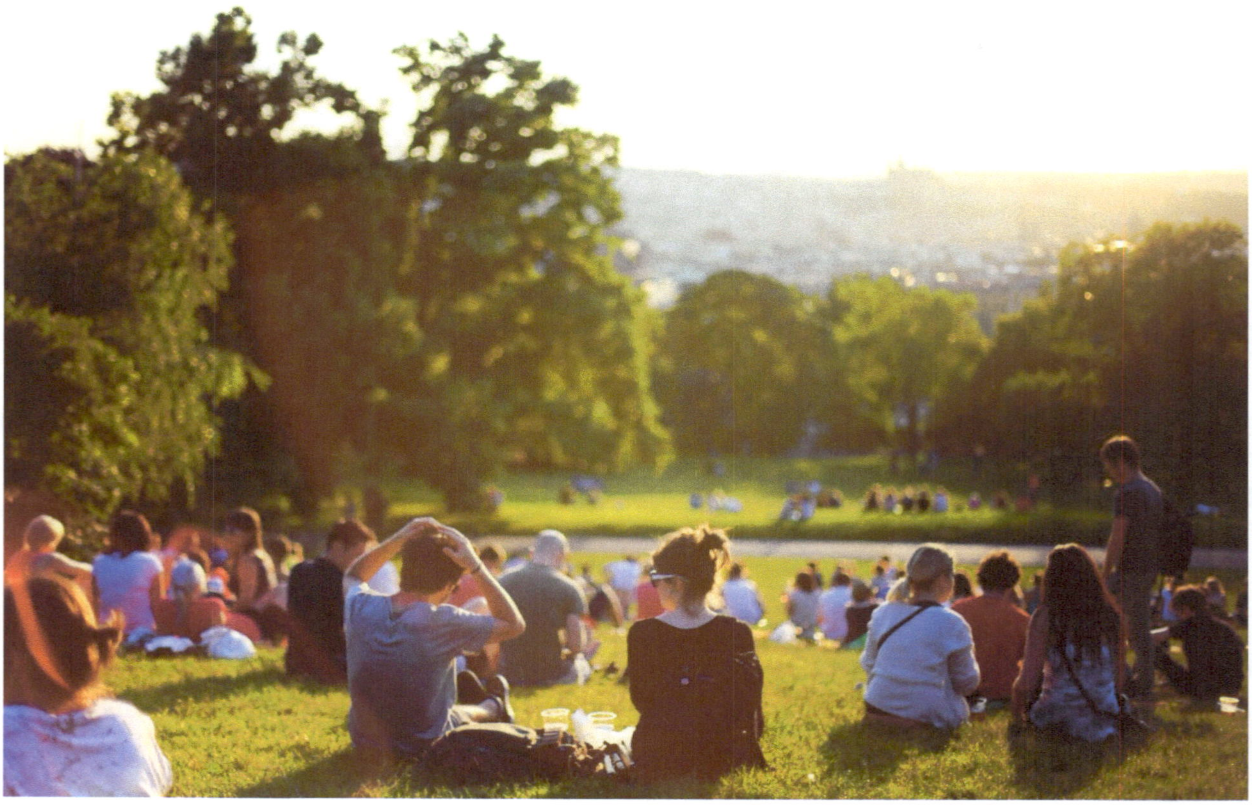

Nurturing and sustaining community connections requires regular participation and engagement. Attend group activities consistently, whether they're weekly meetings, monthly workshops, or casual coffee catch-ups. These regular interactions help maintain the bonds you've formed and keep you anchored to a network that supports your growth and well-being. Building a personal support network within these broader communities can provide more focused assistance. Identify individuals you connect with on a deeper level and reach out to them. Whether it's a small group you meet with regularly or a few friends you call on tough days, a personal support network offers tailored encouragement and accountability. These relationships thrive on mutual respect and understanding, growing stronger through shared experiences and ongoing communication.

As we wrap up this chapter, remember that your community is more than a lifeline; it's a source of strength and solidarity. By finding your tribe, contributing to shared growth, and nurturing these connections, you build a foundation of support that enriches your life. This chapter has explored how nurturing relationships, whether through clear communication, conflict resolution, or community engagement, can significantly enhance your experience with ADHD. Next, we will explore strategies for financial literacy, ensuring you have the tools to manage your resources effectively.

CHAPTER 5
FINANCIAL LITERACY FOR THE ADHD MIND

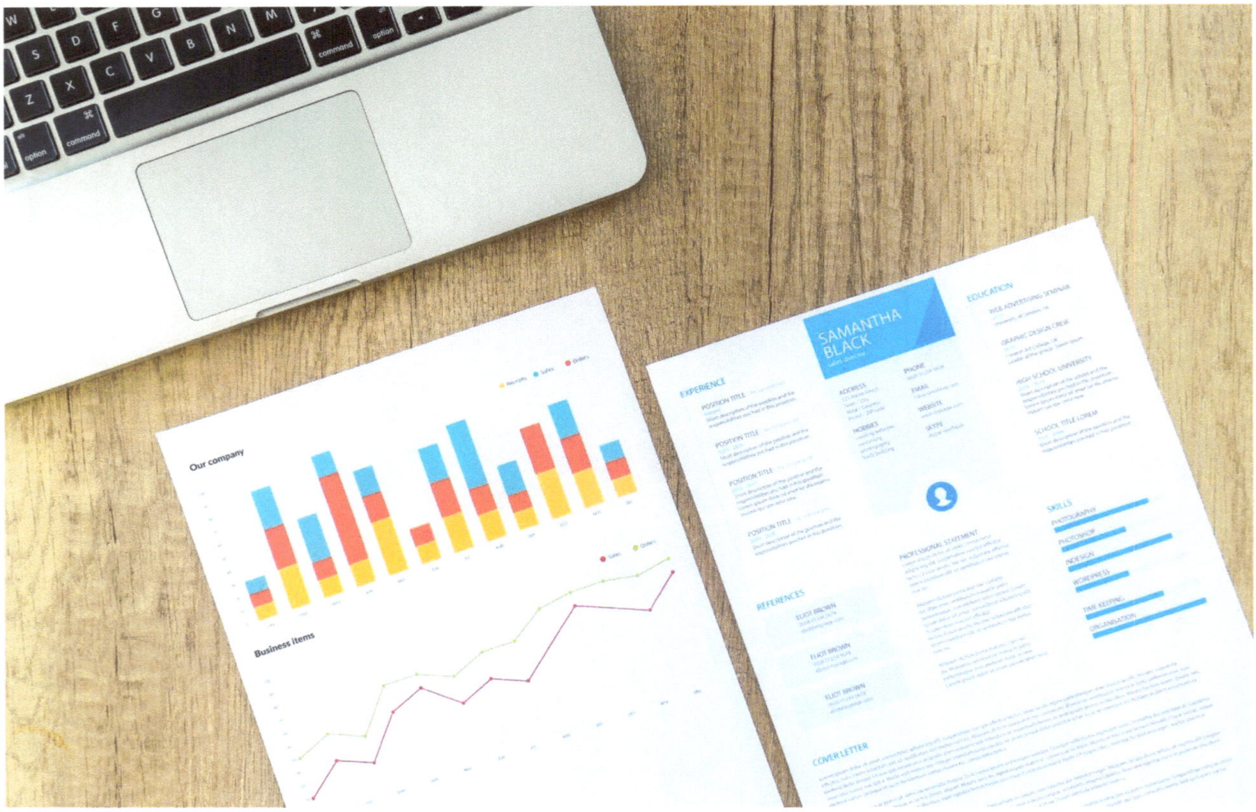

I USED to think budgeting was like trying to solve a Rubik's cube in the dark. I once sat at my kitchen table, surrounded by stacks of unopened bills and receipts, feeling like I was drowning in a sea of numbers and obligations. My ADHD brain craved structure, yet the idea of creating a budget seemed overwhelming and tedious. That's when I realized that budgeting isn't just about math — it's a roadmap for your financial journey, guiding you toward stability and peace of mind. It helps you track your spending, identify patterns, and make informed decisions about your money. Budgeting is your compass, pointing you toward your financial goals and helping you avoid the pitfalls of impulsive spending and financial stress.

Creating a simple budget is the first step toward regaining control over your finances. Start by gathering all your financial information, such as bank statements, bills, and receipts. This process might feel daunting, but it's essential for understanding your financial landscape. Once you have everything in front of you, categorize your expenses into needs and wants. Needs include essential expenses like rent, utilities, and groceries, while wants cover non-essential items like dining out or entertainment. This distinction helps you prioritize your spending and allocate your funds effectively. Consider using a budgeting app like You Need a Budget (YNAB), which uses a zero-based budgeting method that assigns every dollar to a job. This app can be a game-changer, offering a structured approach to managing your finances, though it might take some time to get used to.

For those of us with ADHD, traditional budgeting techniques might not always fit. Adapting your budgeting process to accommodate ADHD tendencies can make it more manageable and less stressful. One effective strategy is color-coding your budget categories. Use different colors to highlight various expenses, making it easier to visualize and track your spending. This visual aid can help you stay organized and quickly identify areas where you might be overspending. Setting up automated reminders for bills is another crucial step. Schedule notifications on your phone or use an app to remind you of upcoming due dates. This automation reduces the risk of late payments and keeps your financial obligations at the forefront of your mind. These tools can provide a quick snapshot of your financial health, allowing you to see where your money is going at a glance.

Staying on track with your budget requires consistency and a proactive approach. Weekly budget check-ins can be a powerful tool for maintaining control over your finances. Set aside time each week to review your spending, update your budget, and assess your progress toward your financial goals. This practice not only keeps you accountable but also helps you catch any potential issues before they become significant problems. Life is unpredictable, and your financial situation can change in an instant. Whether it's a job change, a new expense, or a shift in income, be prepared to adjust your budget accordingly. Flexibility is key to successful budgeting, allowing you to adapt to changing circumstances without losing sight of your financial objectives.

Interactive Element: Budget Reflection Exercise

Reflect on your current budgeting habits. Consider the following questions: What challenges do you face when trying to stick to a budget? Are there specific categories where you tend to overspend? How do you feel about your current financial situation? Write down your thoughts and identify one or two areas where you can make improvements. This reflection is an opportunity to gain insight into your financial habits and develop a more effective budgeting strategy tailored to your needs.

By embracing these ADHD-friendly budgeting techniques, you can transform the way you manage your finances. Rather than feeling overwhelmed, you'll gain a sense of empowerment and control, turning budgeting into a tool that supports your financial well-being.

SAVINGS GOALS: BUILDING YOUR FINANCIAL FUTURE

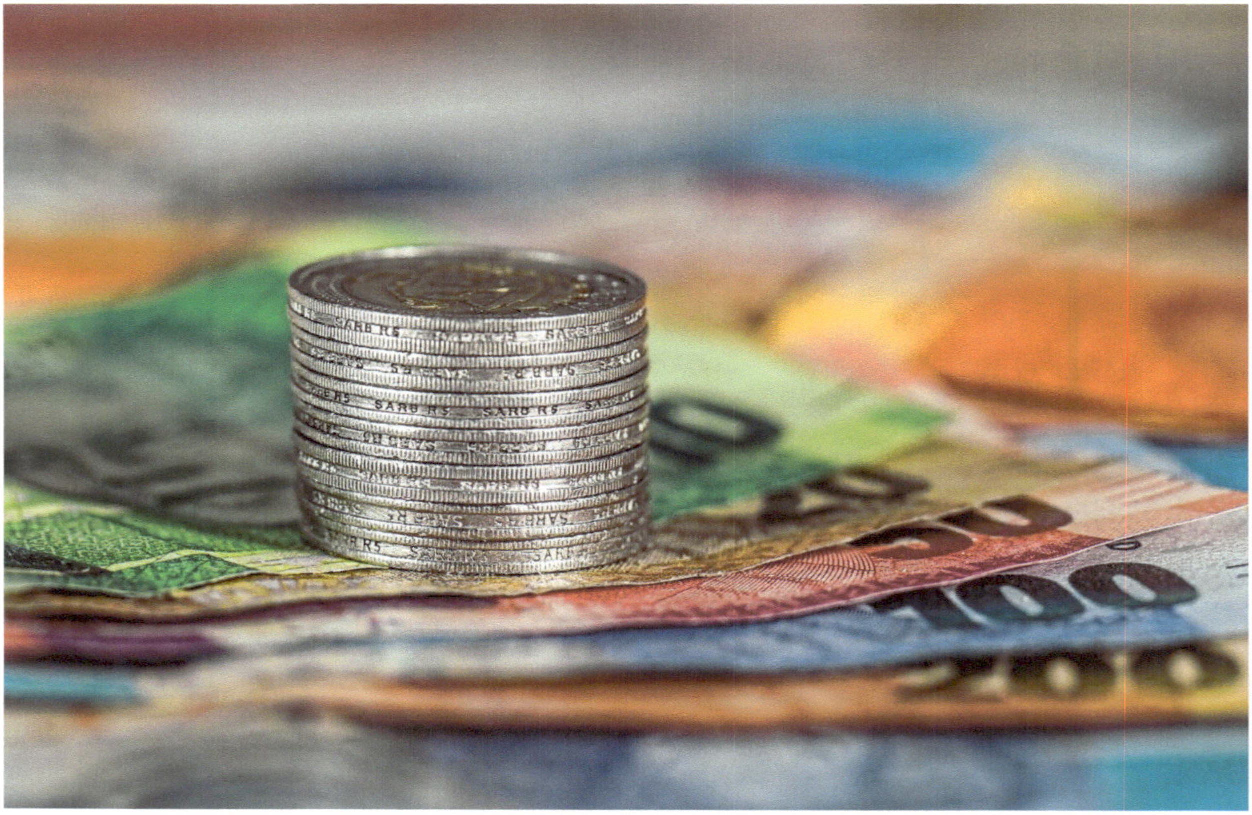

When thinking about savings goals, it can feel like standing at the base of a mountain, unsure of where to start climbing. The key is to break it down into manageable steps. Begin by defining your short-term and long-term savings goals. Short-term goals might include saving for a new gadget or a holiday, while long-term goals could be buying a home or building a retirement fund.

To make these goals more tangible, consider creating a vision board. This visual representation of your financial objectives can serve as a constant reminder of where you're headed. Stick images or words on a board that symbolize your goals, and place it somewhere you see daily, like your workspace or bedroom. This not only keeps your goals in the forefront of your mind but also helps prioritize them based on urgency and importance. By having a clear picture of what you want to achieve, you can allocate your resources accordingly and stay focused on what truly matters.

Once your goals are set, the next step is to develop strategies for consistent saving. Consistency is crucial because it transforms saving from an occasional effort into a regular habit. One effective method is automating your savings transfers. Set up automatic transfers from your checking account to your savings account right after you receive your paycheck. This ensures that a portion of your income is saved before you have a chance to spend it — it's like paying yourself first.

Another helpful approach is using apps that round up your purchases to the nearest dollar and deposit the difference into your savings account. This small change, which you might not even notice, can add up over time, gradually increasing your savings without feeling like a burden. These strategies help build a savings routine that requires minimal effort yet delivers significant results.

Building an emergency fund is another critical aspect of securing your financial future. This fund acts as a safety net, providing financial security when unexpected expenses arise, such as medical bills or car repairs. It's important to set a specific target for your emergency fund, typically covering three to six months' worth of living expenses. This amount might seem daunting at first, but it's achievable with small, consistent contributions. Start by setting aside a manageable amount each month, even if it's just a small percentage of your income. Over time, these contributions will accumulate, creating a buffer against financial surprises. Remember, the goal is progress, not perfection, and every little bit helps in building that safety net.

Staying motivated and accountable to your savings goals can sometimes be challenging, especially when life throws unexpected curveballs. Finding a savings buddy can be a game-changer. This person could be a friend or family member with similar financial goals. By partnering up, you can encourage each other, share tips, and celebrate milestones together. This mutual support system creates a sense of accountability, making it harder to stray from your goals.

Celebrating milestones is another powerful motivator. When you reach a savings target, reward yourself with a non-monetary treat, like a day off to relax or a special outing. Recognizing and celebrating your achievements reinforces positive behavior and keeps you motivated to continue saving.

DEBT MANAGEMENT: STRATEGIES FOR SUCCESS

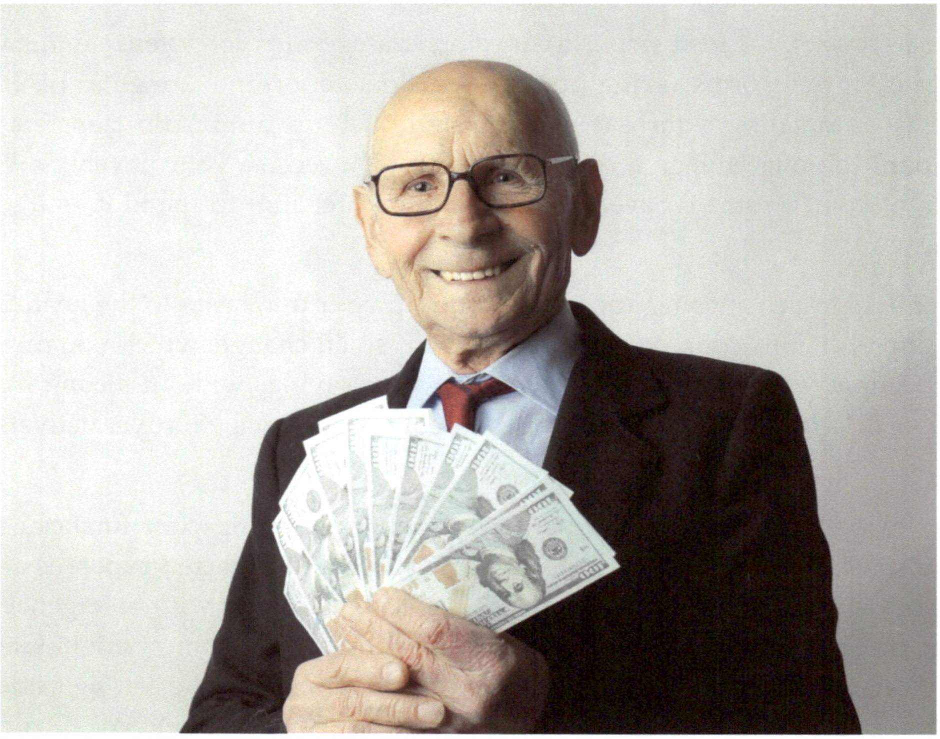

Understanding debt can feel like untangling a ball of yarn, with each thread representing a different financial commitment. Not all debt is created equal, and recognizing the difference between good and bad debt is crucial for your financial health. Good debt, like student loans, is often considered an investment in your future. It can lead to higher earning potential and career advancement, justifying the initial financial burden. Also, your debts for your self-employed business are good as well. You can use these expenses to offset your taxes. On the other hand, credit card debt is typically seen as bad debt, especially when it accumulates due to high interest rates and impulsive spending. It's the kind of debt that can spiral out of control if not managed carefully, trapping you in a cycle of minimum payments and growing balances. Interest rates play a significant role in this dynamic. The higher the rate, the longer it takes to pay off the debt and the more you end up paying in the long run. Understanding these nuances helps you navigate your financial landscape with greater awareness and control.

Creating a debt repayment plan is like mapping out a strategy for climbing a mountain. You need a clear path and a set of tools to reach the summit. Two popular methods for tackling debt are the snowball and avalanche methods. The snowball method involves paying off your smallest debts first, gaining momentum and confidence with each cleared balance. This psychological boost can be motivating, helping you tackle larger debts with renewed determination. In contrast, the avalanche method focuses on paying off debts with the highest interest rates first, saving you more money over time. Both approaches have their merits, and the choice depends on your financial situation and personal preferences. Prioritizing high-interest debts is often a wise strategy, as it reduces the overall cost of borrowing and shortens the repayment period. By focusing on these debts, you can free up more resources to address other financial goals.

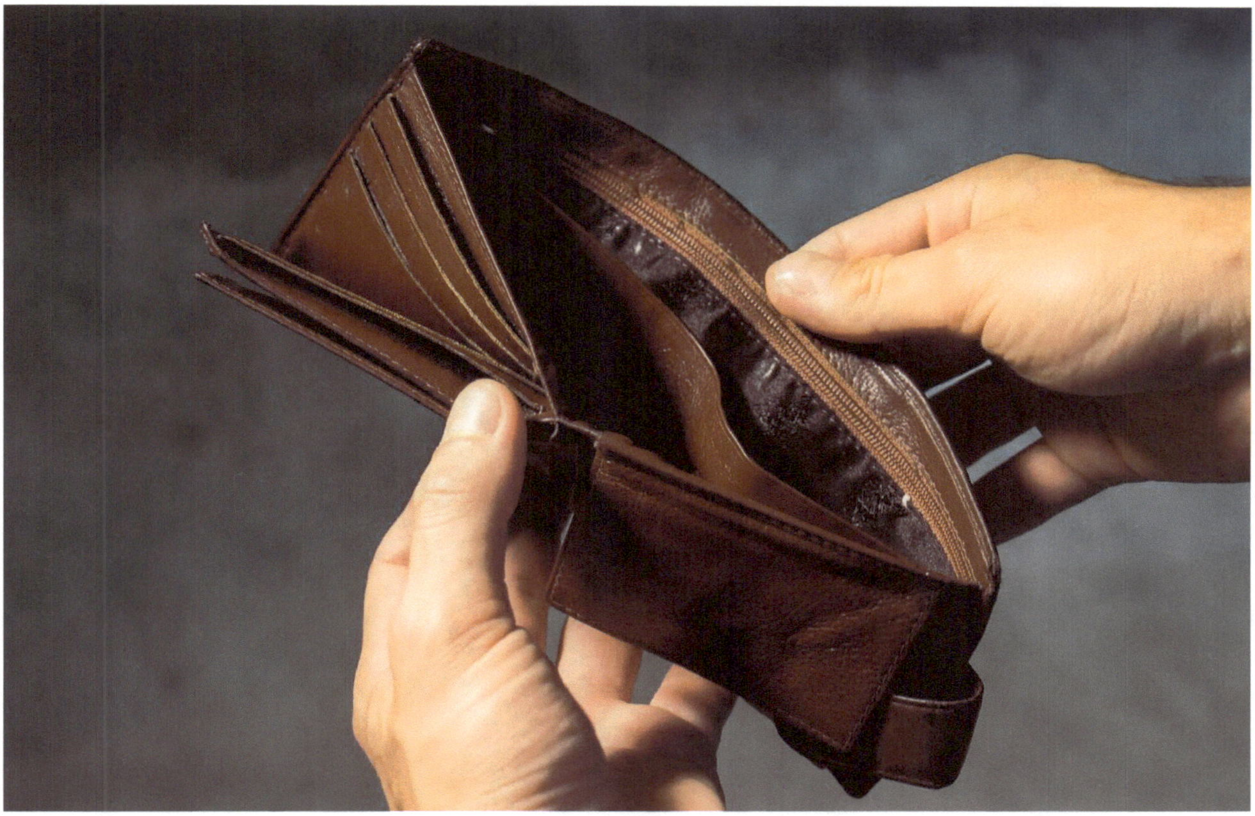

Avoiding common debt traps is essential to maintaining your financial well-being. Compulsive spending is a significant pitfall, often driven by emotional triggers or a desire for instant gratification. Recognizing the signs of this behavior, such as frequent impulse purchases or buying items you don't need, can help you take control. Setting limits on credit card usage is another critical step. Only use your card for planned expenses, and pay off the balance in full each month to avoid accumulating interest. These practices help you develop a healthier relationship with spending, reducing the likelihood of falling into debt. It's about being mindful of your financial decisions and understanding the long-term impact they can have.

Resources for debt management assistance are abundant, offering support and guidance to help you regain control. Credit counseling services provide personalized advice and strategies for managing debt, often free of charge or at a low cost. These professionals can help you create a budget, negotiate with creditors, and develop a realistic repayment plan. Online debt management tools, like calculators and budget planners, offer additional support, allowing you to track your progress and stay accountable. Utilizing these resources empowers you to take charge of your financial situation, transforming debt from a source of stress into a manageable challenge.

Debt doesn't have to be an insurmountable obstacle. With the right strategies and support, you can navigate the complexities of debt management and work toward financial stability. By understanding the nature of your debt, creating a plan, and using available resources, you can make informed decisions that align with your financial goals. This proactive approach not only alleviates financial stress but also sets the stage for a more secure and prosperous future.

FINANCIAL PLANNING: TURNING DREAMS INTO REALITY

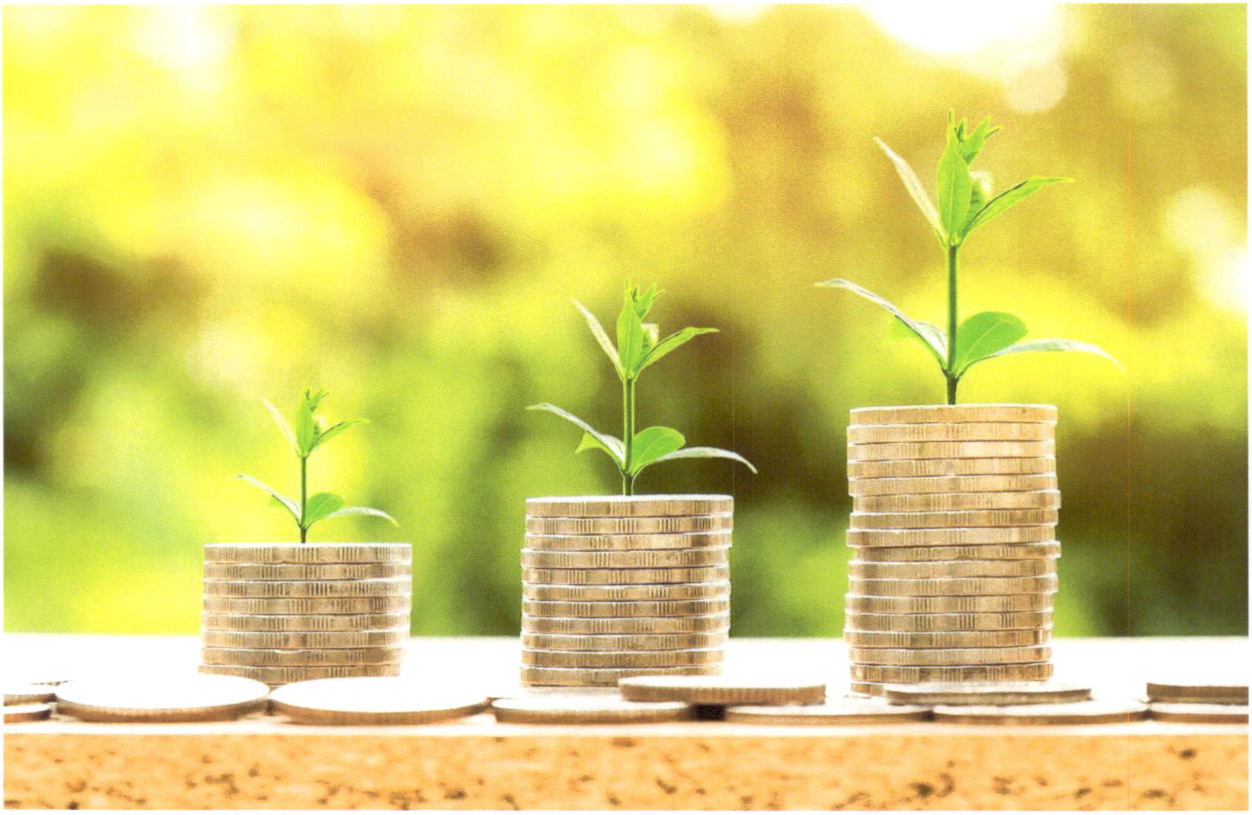

Setting financial goals can often feel overwhelming, like staring at a blank canvas, unsure where to place the first brushstroke. But the process doesn't have to be daunting. It begins with envisioning what you want your financial future to look like. Perhaps it's owning a cozy home, traveling the world, or simply enjoying a comfortable retirement without financial stress. Once you have this vision, break it down into manageable steps. Start by identifying short-term goals, which might include paying off a small debt or saving for a vacation, and align them with long-term aspirations, such as building a retirement fund. By balancing these desires, you ensure that immediate pleasures don't overshadow future security, allowing you to allocate resources wisely and stay motivated. Setting clear, actionable steps for each goal creates a roadmap that guides your financial decisions, turning abstract wishes into achievable targets.

Creating a personal financial plan is like constructing a building—each element must fit together to form a stable structure. Begin by incorporating investments and savings into your overall strategy. Determine how much you can realistically set aside each month for savings and how much you can allocate to investments. Diversifying your investment portfolio is crucial; it reduces risk by spreading your money across various asset classes like stocks, bonds, and real estate. Consider consulting with a financial advisor to explore options that align with your risk tolerance and financial goals. Investments aren't just about the potential to grow your wealth; they represent a commitment to your future, a step toward financial independence. Regularly reviewing and adjusting your financial plan is equally important. Life is unpredictable, and your financial needs may shift as circumstances change. Make it a point to assess your plan at least annually, adjusting for any major life changes or evolving goals. This flexibility ensures your financial strategy remains relevant and effective, adapting to life's twists and turns with confidence.

Building wealth over time requires patience and a strategic approach. One of the most powerful tools at your disposal is the concept of compound interest. This is where your money earns interest, and then that interest earns interest, creating a snowball effect that grows your wealth exponentially over time. The earlier you start investing, the more you benefit from this compounding effect. Even small, consistent contributions can lead to substantial growth if given enough time. Understanding this principle can transform your approach to saving and investing, highlighting the value of starting early and staying consistent. It's about planting seeds now and nurturing them, allowing them to bloom into a flourishing financial garden.

Securing your financial future involves preparing for significant life events with foresight and planning. Retirement might seem distant, but it's never too early to start planning for it. Contribute regularly to retirement accounts like a 401(k) or IRA, taking advantage of any employer matching programs to maximize your savings potential. These contributions offer tax advantages and compound over the years, providing a steady income stream when you're ready to retire. If you have children, saving for their education is another crucial consideration. Explore savings plans like 529 accounts, which offer tax benefits and can significantly offset future educational expenses. Education is one of the best gifts you can give, as it provides opportunities and opens doors.

Additionally, consider purchasing insurance to protect against unexpected events. Health, life, and disability insurance offer peace of mind, safeguarding your financial stability against unforeseen circumstances. These measures not only protect your assets but also provide a safety net, allowing you to navigate life's uncertainties with greater confidence and security.

Financial planning is about more than just numbers; it's about crafting a life that aligns with your values and dreams. By setting clear goals, creating a flexible plan, and preparing for the future, you lay the foundation for financial stability and success. This chapter has explored the process of turning your financial aspirations into reality, emphasizing the importance of planning and adaptability. As we move forward, we'll delve into career development strategies, focusing on how to align your professional path with your financial and personal goals.

REVIEW REQUEST FOR ADHD LIFE SKILLS 101

As a therapist and someone who lives with ADHD, I know how it feels to have a brain that's always on the go. One minute, you're stuck staring at a to-do list that feels impossible, and the next, you're coming up with brilliant ideas that surprise even yourself. I'll never forget the day I was drowning in paperwork, feeling like I couldn't keep up, when a client walked in, beaming with pride over a breakthrough we'd worked on together. In that moment, I realized my ADHD wasn't holding me back—it was helping me connect with others in ways I never imagined. That's why I wrote *ADHD Life Skills 101*.

This book is your go-to guide for understanding ADHD and turning it into your superpower. Whether you're a parent trying to support your child, a therapist looking for new tools, or someone with ADHD seeking self-improvement, this book is here to help. It's packed with practical tips, emotional support strategies, and insights to help you see ADHD in a whole new light.

If you've read *ADHD Life Skills 101*, I'd love to hear your thoughts! Your review can help others discover how this book can make a difference in their lives. Here are a few things you could share in your review:

- What did you learn about ADHD that surprised you?

- How has this book helped you or someone you care about?

- Which strategies or tips have you found most useful?

Your feedback means the world to me, and it helps others find the support they need. Thank you for being part of this journey to transform how we see and live with ADHD!

Click here to leave your review!

[Insert link to review platform]

https://www.amazon.com/review/review-your-purchases/?asin=BOOKASIN

With gratitude,

Jamaal Simmons, LCSW-C

Author of *ADHD Life Skills 101*

CHAPTER 6
CAREER DEVELOPMENT STRATEGIES

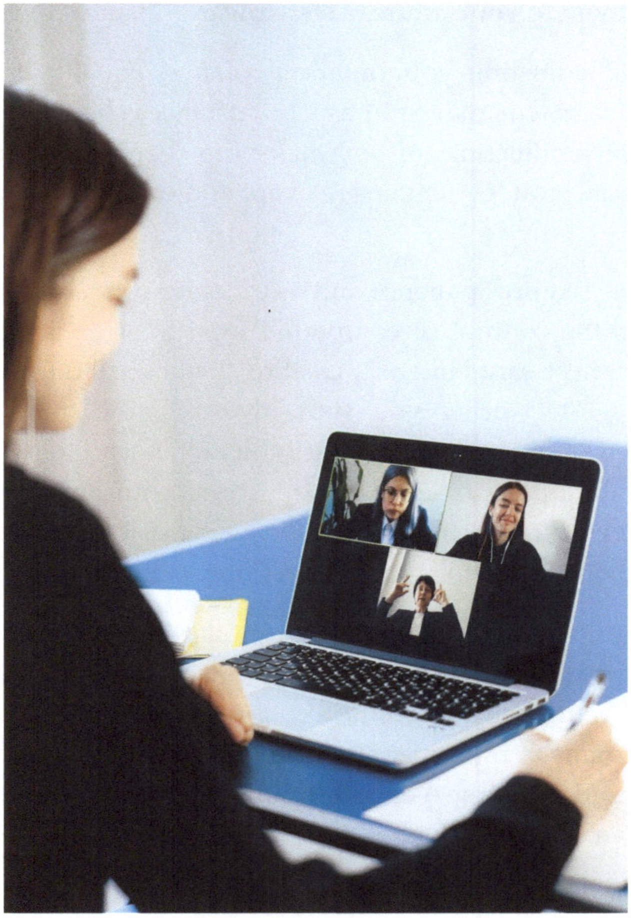

SETTING financial goals can often feel overwhelming, like staring at a blank canvas, unsure where to place the first brushstroke. But the process doesn't have to be daunting. It begins with envisioning what you want your financial future to look like. Perhaps it's owning a cozy home, traveling the world, or simply enjoying a comfortable retirement without financial stress. Once you have this vision, break it down into manageable steps. Start by identifying short-term goals, which might include paying off a small debt or saving for a vacation, and align them with long-term aspirations, such as building a retirement fund. By balancing these desires, you ensure that immediate pleasures don't overshadow future security, allowing you to allocate resources wisely and stay motivated. Setting clear, actionable steps for each goal creates a roadmap that guides your financial decisions, turning abstract wishes into achievable targets.

Creating a personal financial plan is like constructing a building—each element must fit together to form a stable structure. Begin by incorporating investments and savings into your overall strategy. Determine how much you can realistically set aside each month for savings and how much you can allocate to investments. Diversifying your investment portfolio is crucial; it reduces risk by spreading your money across various asset classes like stocks, bonds, and real estate. Consider consulting with a financial advisor to explore options that align with your risk tolerance and financial goals. Investments aren't just about the potential to grow your wealth; they represent a commitment to your future, a step toward financial independence.

Regularly reviewing and adjusting your financial plan is equally important. Life is unpredictable, and your financial needs may shift as circumstances change. Make it a point to assess your plan at least annually, adjusting for any major life changes or evolving goals. This flexibility ensures your financial strategy remains relevant and effective, adapting to life's twists and turns with confidence.

Building wealth over time requires patience and a strategic approach. One of the most powerful tools at your disposal is the concept of compound interest. This is where your money earns interest, and then that interest earns interest, creating a snowball effect that grows your wealth exponentially over time. The earlier you start investing, the more you benefit from this compounding effect. Even small, consistent contributions can lead to substantial growth if given enough time. Understanding this principle can transform your approach to saving and investing, highlighting the value of starting early and staying consistent. It's about planting seeds now and nurturing them, allowing them to bloom into a flourishing financial garden.

Securing your financial future involves preparing for significant life events with foresight and planning. Retirement might seem distant, but it's never too early to start planning for it. Contribute regularly to retirement accounts like a 401(k) or IRA, taking advantage of any employer matching programs to maximize your savings potential. These contributions offer tax advantages and compound over the years, providing a steady income stream when you're ready to retire. If you have children, save for their future.

I remember the first time I thought seriously about my career. I was sitting in a coffee shop, laptop open, staring at a blank document titled "Future Plans?" It felt like trying to map out a journey without a destination. The possibilities were endless, but the path was unclear. It was both exhilarating and daunting, especially with ADHD adding its own layer of complexity. My thoughts raced between ideas, each one sparking a different direction. What I needed was a way to focus that energy, to harness it into something tangible and productive. That's when I realized the importance of truly understanding my strengths and aspirations.

Identifying personal strengths can be a bit like peeling an onion. Each layer reveals something new, and sometimes it brings tears. For many of us, understanding our strengths isn't straightforward. We've often been told what we're not good at but are rarely encouraged to explore what we excel in. Self-assessment tools like the Clifton-Strengths assessment can be a game-changer here. This tool helps pinpoint your core strengths by highlighting key themes that define how you naturally think, feel, and behave. Reflecting on past successes and achievements is another powerful method. Think about moments when you felt most alive when your work felt effortless. These are often clues to your underlying strengths. Consider asking friends or colleagues for their observations, as they might see strengths you take for granted. By embracing these exercises, you begin to paint a clearer picture of what makes you you.

Once you've identified your strengths, the next step is alignment—mapping these strengths to potential career paths. This is where the magic happens, where you connect what you love with what you do. For those with ADHD, it's about finding industries that appreciate traits like creativity and problem-solving. Marketing is a good example, where the fast-paced, dynamic environment thrives on innovation and adaptability, qualities many with ADHD naturally possess. But don't limit yourself to traditional roles. Consider emerging new industries that value diversity of thought and unconventional approaches. Aligning your strengths with career goals isn't about fitting into a mold; it's about finding a place where your unique abilities shine. Research different fields, talk to people in those roles, and imagine yourself in those scenarios.

Setting career goals can feel overwhelming, like standing at the base of a mountain and trying to see the peak. But breaking it down into manageable steps can make it achievable. This is where SMART goals come in—specific, measurable, achievable, relevant, and time-bound objectives. Start with short-term goals, like acquiring a new skill or networking with professionals in your field. These are the footholds that will help you climb higher. Then, envision your long-term aspirations. What does success look like to you? What kind of impact do you want to have? Visioning exercises can help here. Create a vision board or write a letter to your future self describing your ideal career and life. This not only clarifies your goals but fuels your motivation to pursue them.

Self-doubt is a familiar companion in the goal-setting process, often whispering that you're not good enough or that success is out of reach. It's important to acknowledge these feelings but not let them dictate your path. Affirmations can reinforce self-belief, acting as a counter to the negative narrative. Repeating phrases like "I am capable" or "I have the skills to succeed" can gradually shift your mindset. Mentorship also plays a vital role in building confidence. A mentor provides guidance, shares their experiences, and offers a different perspective on your challenges. They can help you see beyond your doubts, encouraging you to take risks and celebrate your progress. Surrounding yourself with supportive voices creates a buffer against self-doubt, allowing you to focus on your growth.

Interactive Element: Strengths and Aspirations Worksheet

Take a moment to jot down your top five strengths. Next to each strength, list at least two career paths or industries that might value those skills. Consider what excites you about these paths and how they align with your long-term aspirations. Reflect on any obstacles you perceive and brainstorm ways to overcome them. This exercise helps ground your career development in a clear understanding of your strengths and aspirations, setting the stage for meaningful progress.

Let's embrace the unique traits that ADHD brings to the table and use them as stepping stones to success.

NETWORKING FOR PROFESSIONAL GROWTH

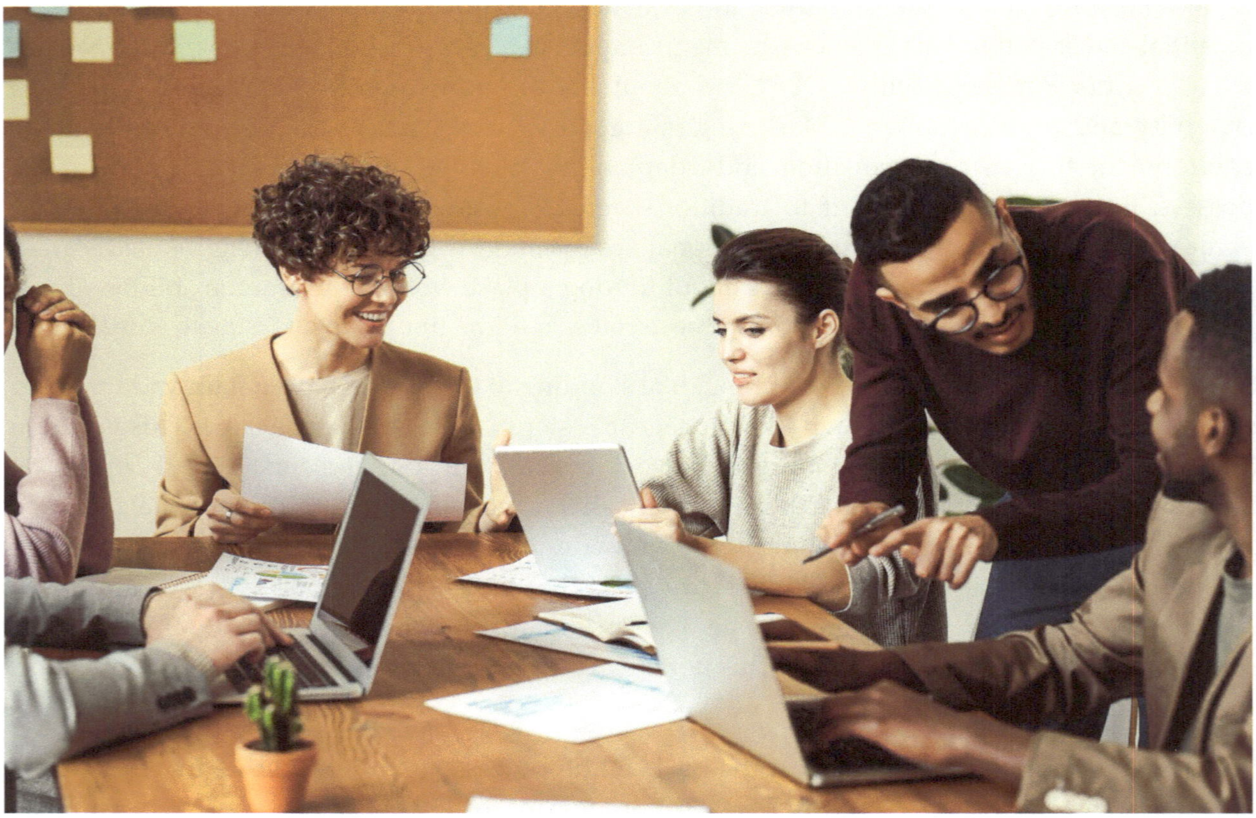

Networking has always felt like a bit of an exhausting maze to me. It's this intricate dance where you meet people, share a bit about yourself, and try to build connections that could lead to something more. For those of us with ADHD, the idea of networking can be both thrilling and daunting. It is thrilling because of the endless possibilities it offers, but it is also daunting because it involves navigating social cues, remembering names, and following up—all while trying to stay focused. But here's the thing: networking is crucial for career advancement. It's about building relationships that provide support and open doors to new opportunities. Think of it as planting seeds in a garden; each interaction is a seed that, with care, can grow into something fruitful.

Building relationships through networking is not just about what others can do for you. It's a two-way street where you offer your own insights, skills, and support in return. This reciprocity is where the real magic happens. When you connect with people from different backgrounds and industries, you expand your knowledge and perspectives. Diverse connections challenge your thinking, introduce you to new ideas, and can even inspire you to take paths you hadn't considered before. It's like having a personal think tank at your fingertips, ready to brainstorm and solve problems with you. And in this ever-evolving professional landscape, having a network of people who can offer advice and feedback is invaluable.

For those of us navigating the complexities of ADHD, effective networking strategies require a bit of planning and creativity. One of the most useful tools in your networking arsenal is the elevator pitch. Imagine you're in an elevator with someone you admire, and you only have a few floors to introduce yourself and make an impression. Crafting a concise, compelling pitch helps you articulate who you are and what you're looking for. Practice it until it feels natural and confident.

Online platforms like LinkedIn are also fantastic for professional networking. They allow you to connect with people globally, join industry groups, and participate in discussions. The key is to be proactive—reach out to people who inspire you, ask questions, and engage with their content. It might feel intimidating at first, but you'll find that most people appreciate genuine connection.

Building and maintaining these relationships over time is where the real work begins. It's not enough to meet people; you need to nurture those connections. Regular follow-ups are a simple yet effective way to stay on someone's radar. Whether it's a quick message to check in, share an article you think they'd enjoy, or congratulate them on a recent achievement, these small gestures show that you value the relationship.

Offering value before asking for help is another crucial strategy. Consider what you can contribute to the relationship—maybe it's sharing a resource, offering a skill, or simply being a sounding board. By giving first, you create a foundation of trust and reciprocity, making it more likely that others will want to help you in return.

Then there are networking events, those bustling gatherings that can be both exciting and nerve-wracking. For those with ADHD, managing the social anxiety that often accompanies these events is key. One strategy is to set specific goals for each event. Maybe you want to meet three new people, learn about a specific topic, or connect with someone from a particular company. Having these goals gives you a sense of purpose and can help focus your attention amidst the chaos.

It's also perfectly okay to take breaks if you feel overwhelmed. Step outside for a breath of fresh air, or find a quiet corner to recharge. Remember, quality trumps quantity. It's better to have a few meaningful conversations than to collect a stack of business cards with no real connections.

Networking is not just about business cards and LinkedIn connections. It's about genuine relationships that enrich your career and personal growth. By approaching networking with authenticity, curiosity, and a willingness to contribute, you'll find that it becomes less of a chore and more of an opportunity. It's about finding your tribe and building a community that supports and challenges you.

OVERCOMING IMPOSTER SYNDROME

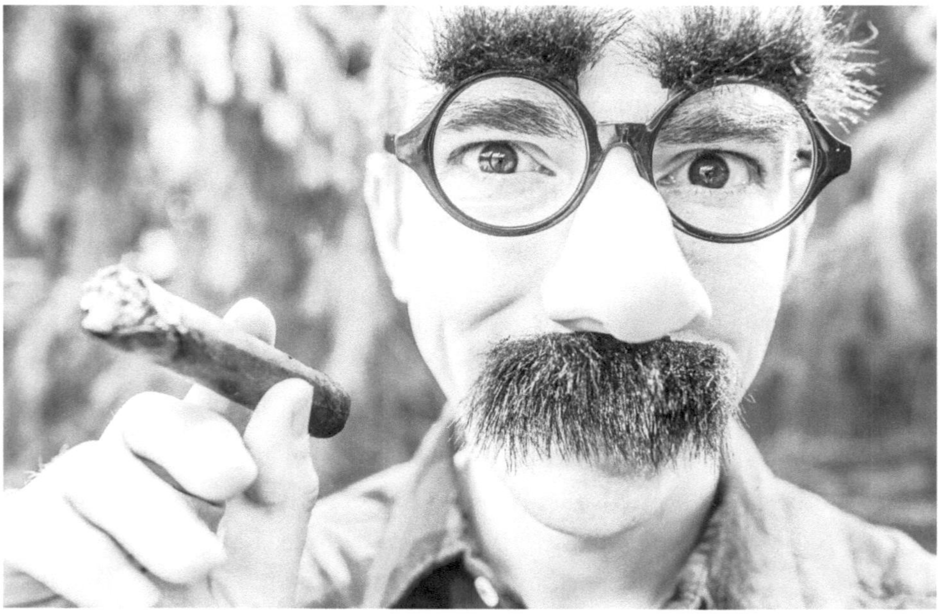

Imposter syndrome is a sneaky beast. It's that nagging voice in the back of your mind questioning your achievements, whispering doubts about your worth, and convincing you that you're a fraud. Even when you're standing on the mountain of your accomplishments, it insists you're about to be unmasked. For those of us with ADHD, this cycle of self-doubt can be particularly vicious. ADHD traits like forgetfulness, impulsivity, and the struggle to focus can amplify feelings of inadequacy. The irony is that while ADHD can fuel creativity and innovation, it can also make us feel like we're perpetually falling short, no matter how much we achieve. It's a cruel twist, isn't it? You're thriving in your career, yet there's a part of you bracing for the moment someone points and says, "You don't belong here."

Recognizing when you're caught in the grip of imposter syndrome is the first step toward breaking free. The signs are often subtle but consistent. Do you find yourself downplaying your accomplishments, attributing them to luck or the help of others rather than your own skills? Maybe you live in fear of being exposed as a fraud, always waiting for the other shoe to drop. Keeping a journal can be incredibly revealing here. Start jotting down moments when these thoughts creep in. What triggered them? How did you feel? Over time, patterns will emerge, helping you understand when and why you experience imposter syndrome. This awareness can be eye-opening, as it often highlights how deeply ingrained these feelings are, but it also gives you the power to challenge them.

Once you've identified these feelings, combating imposter syndrome involves a mix of strategies. Cognitive restructuring is a fancy term for changing how you think. It involves challenging those negative beliefs and replacing them with more realistic, positive ones. When that voice in your head tells you, "You're not good enough," counter it with, "I've achieved this because I'm skilled and capable." It sounds simple, but with practice, it becomes a powerful tool for shifting your mindset. Celebrating successes, no matter how small, is another key strategy. Take time to acknowledge your skills and achievements. Write them down, share them with a friend, or even treat yourself to something special. This isn't about bragging; it's about reminding yourself of your value. Seeking feedback from colleagues or mentors can also provide a more objective perspective on your abilities. A mentor, in particular, can offer guidance and reassurance, helping you see your strengths through a clearer lens.

Building self-efficacy, or belief in your capabilities, is crucial for overcoming imposter syndrome. Start by setting incremental challenges that push you slightly out of your comfort zone. These challenges should be just enough to stretch your abilities without overwhelming you. Completing them builds confidence and reinforces your competence. Regular reflection is also important. Make it a habit to look back on your progress, noting how far you've come and what you've learned along the way. Reflecting on your journey (there it is, that word we're not supposed to use) can be incredibly affirming. It's a reminder that you're not just standing still; you're growing and evolving every day.

Imposter syndrome is an insidious companion, but it doesn't have to dictate your narrative. By identifying these feelings, challenging negative beliefs, and building your self-efficacy, you can begin to silence that nagging voice and embrace your achievements with the recognition they deserve. Remember, you're not an imposter. You're exactly where you need to be, and you've earned your place there, even if that little voice sometimes tries to tell you otherwise.

CRAFTING A CAREER ROADMAP

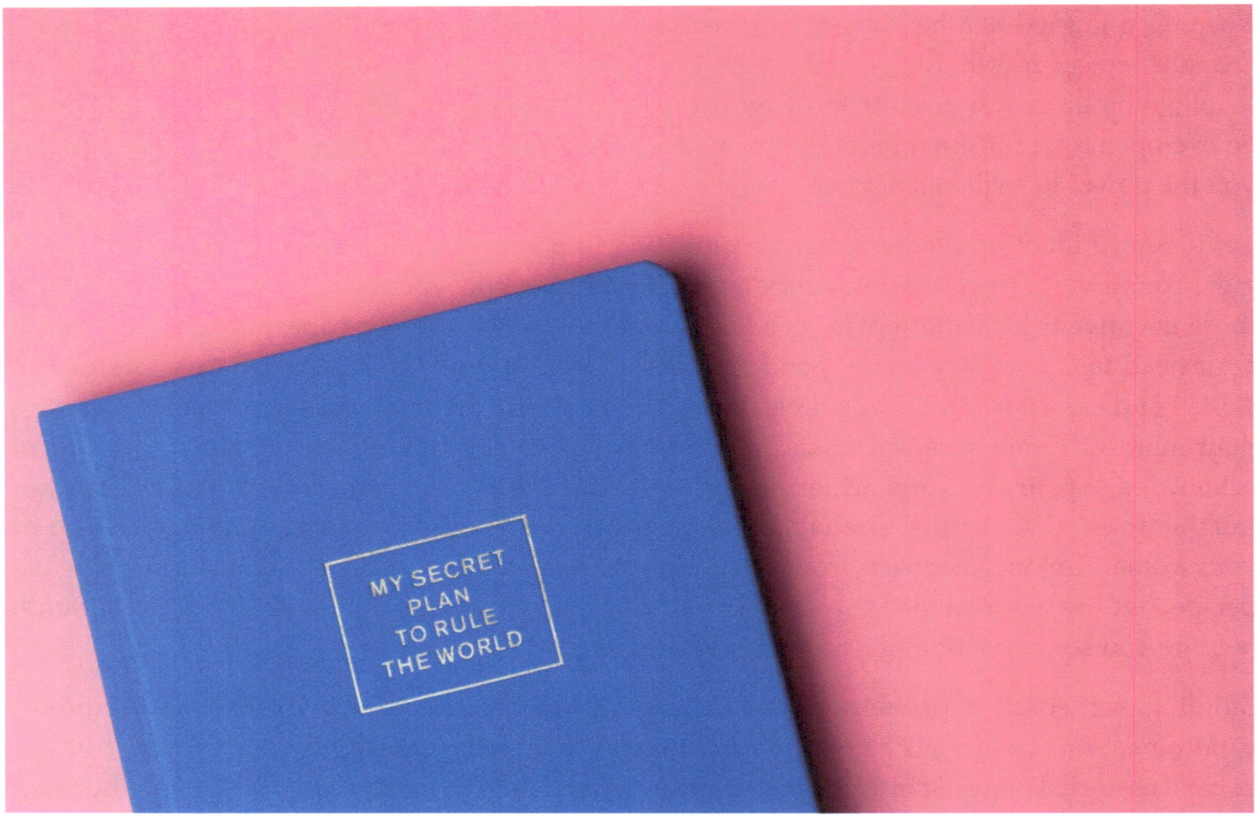

Imagine your career as a road trip. You're not just driving aimlessly; you have destinations in mind, stops along the way, and maybe even a playlist to keep you energized. A career roadmap is essentially your GPS for professional life—it helps you visualize where you want to go and how you'll get there. This roadmap isn't just about reaching the final destination; it's about setting checkpoints that guide your progress and keep you on track. These milestones act like mile markers, letting you know how far you've come and what's still ahead. With a roadmap, you can clearly see your career progression, which not only gives you direction but also helps you stay motivated as you tick off each milestone.

Creating a personalized career roadmap involves a few key steps, starting with identifying your career objectives. Think of these as your ultimate destinations—what do you hope to achieve in your professional life? You might want to become an expert in your field, start your own business, or perhaps transition into a completely new industry. Whatever your goals, jot them down. Once you have a clear sense of where you're headed, it's time to outline the skills and experiences you'll need to get there. Consider what qualifications, certifications, or experiences are necessary. Maybe you need to learn a new software program, gain leadership experience, or even return to school. Aligning these steps with your personal values is crucial. Your roadmap should reflect not just your career objectives but also what matters most to you—whether that's work-life balance, creativity, or making a difference in the world.

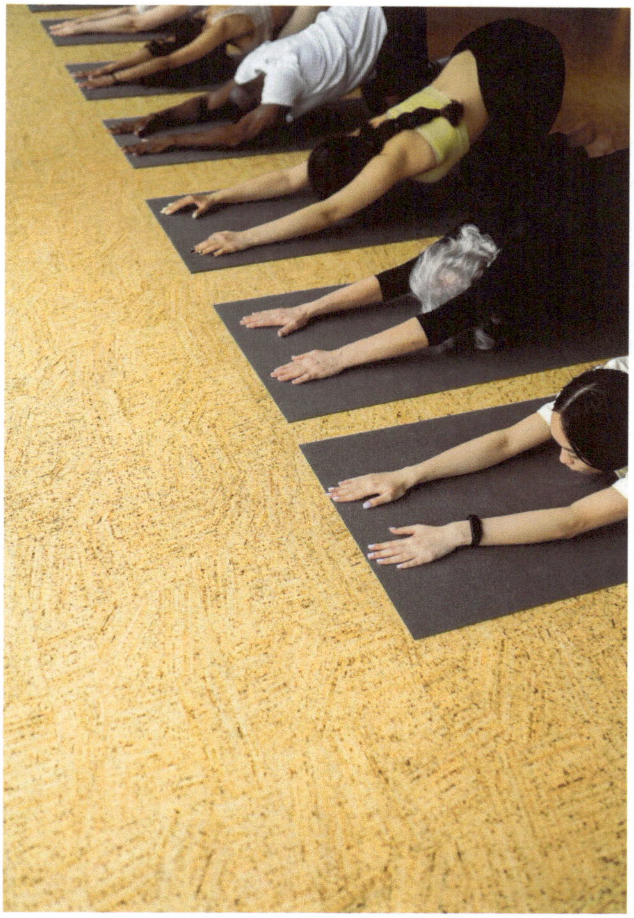

A key component of any effective roadmap is flexibility. Life is unpredictable, and opportunities or challenges can arise unexpectedly. That's why it's important to periodically review and adjust your roadmap. Maybe a new opportunity has come up that aligns perfectly with your skills, or perhaps a change in the industry has shifted your priorities. Regular check-ins with your roadmap allow you to make informed decisions and pivot when necessary. Seeking guidance from career coaches or mentors can provide fresh perspectives and valuable advice. They can help you navigate these changes, offering insights based on their own experiences. Flexibility doesn't mean abandoning your goals; it means adapting your strategies to better suit your evolving path.

A career roadmap isn't just a static document; it's a powerful motivational tool. As you track your achievements and celebrate milestones, you'll gain a sense of accomplishment that fuels your drive to continue. Each milestone you reach is a testament to your progress and resilience. Consider creating visual reminders of your long-term goals—whether it's a vision board, a digital timeline, or a simple list pinned above your desk. These visuals keep your goals in sight, acting as a constant reminder of what you're working towards. They provide motivation on tough days when progress feels slow, reminding you of the bigger picture and helping you push through challenges.

By now, you should have a clearer understanding of how a career roadmap can serve as your personal guide through the professional landscape. It's about setting clear objectives, aligning them with your values, and remaining open to change. As you continue to develop your roadmap, remember that each step you take—no matter how small—is progress. Keep tracking your journey, celebrate your milestones, and stay flexible in your approach. With a well-crafted roadmap, you're not just navigating your career; you're steering it with intention and purpose. This chapter has been a deep dive into career development strategies, equipping you with the tools to move forward confidently. Next, we'll explore how to integrate wellness practices into your professional life, ensuring that your career journey is not only successful but also fulfilling and balanced.

CHAPTER 7
FOSTERING SELF-CARE AND WELLNESS

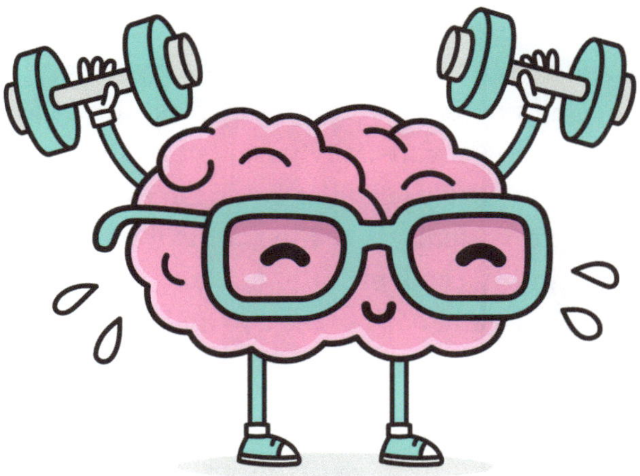

ONE AFTERNOON, I found myself sitting at my desk, surrounded by a steep mountain of tasks, each one clamoring for limited attention. My brain felt like a tangled web of thoughts, each thread pulling me in a different direction. It was then, amid the chaos, that I realized my mind and body were begging for a break. Not just any break, but one that nurtured and restored—a moment of self-care that could quiet the noise and bring clarity. This wasn't just a luxury; it was a necessity. For those of us with ADHD, self-care can act as a lifeline—a way to reclaim focus and manage the restlessness that often accompanies our lives. It's not just about pampering yourself; it's about creating a foundation where mental and physical well-being can thrive.

Understanding the importance of self-care is crucial. It's like refueling a car that's been running on fumes. When your mind is constantly racing, the stress can take a toll, making it difficult to concentrate or maintain emotional balance. Stress reduction is a vital benefit of self-care, allowing your mind to unwind and recharge. When stress is managed, it becomes easier to focus, reducing the scattered thoughts that often derail productivity. Self-care also enhances emotional regulation. By regularly tending to your needs, you create a buffer against the emotional highs and lows that can come with ADHD. This improved regulation helps you respond to situations with calm and composure rather than reacting impulsively.

Creating a personalized self-care routine starts with assessing your personal needs and preferences. It's like curating a playlist that speaks to your soul. Conducting a self-care audit can help identify gaps in your current routine. Take note of activities that bring you joy and relaxation. What makes you feel revived? Is it getting lost in a good book or perhaps a stroll through nature? Exploring different modalities, such as art, music, or spending time outdoors, can reveal what resonates with you. Prioritize activities that spark joy and leave you feeling refreshed, focusing on those that align with your interests and lifestyle. This isn't about fitting into a mold but about creating a routine that feels right for you—something that you'll look forward to instead of seeing as another item on a to-do list.

Once you've identified what works, the next step is designing a routine that fits seamlessly into your lifestyle. It's about weaving self-care into the fabric of your daily life so that it becomes a natural part of your routine rather than a rare indulgence. Time-blocking can be an effective strategy. Set aside specific times for self-care activities, just as you would for important meetings or appointments. This not only ensures that self-care doesn't fall by the wayside but also helps you commit to these practices consistently. Creating a flexible schedule is crucial, particularly for those with ADHD, where rigidity can feel stifling. Allow room for spontaneity and adjust as needed, ensuring that your routine can adapt to the ebb and flow of life's demands.

Monitoring and adjusting your routine is essential to ensure it remains effective. It's like tuning an instrument to keep it playing beautifully. Set monthly check-ins to assess how well your self-care routine is serving you. Are there activities that no longer bring joy, or new interests you'd like to explore? Use these check-ins to make necessary adjustments, ensuring that your routine continues to meet your evolving needs. Keeping a self-care journal can be a valuable tool in this process. Document your experiences, noting what works and what doesn't, and reflect on how these activities impact your well-being. This journal becomes a living guide, helping you fine-tune your approach and keep self-care at the **forefront of your priorities**.

Interactive Element: Self-Care Audit Exercise

Take a moment to conduct a self-care audit. Write down activities that currently make up your self-care routine and evaluate how each one makes you feel. Are there new practices you'd like to try? Reflect on the gaps and opportunities for growth in your self-care journey. Use this audit as a foundation to build a routine that truly nourishes your mind and body.

NUTRITION AND ADHD: FUELING YOUR BRAIN

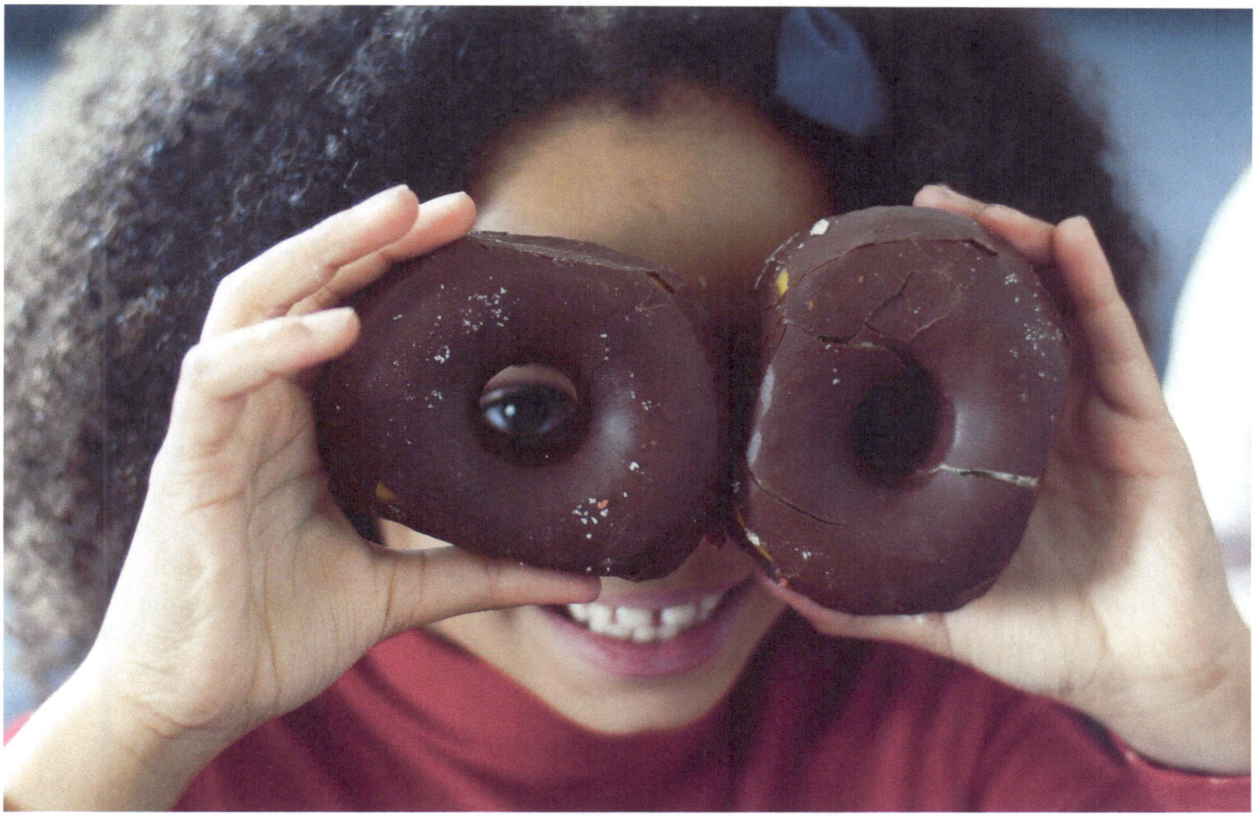

What you put in your body significantly impacts how your brain functions, particularly for those navigating life with ADHD. It's more than just eating to stave off hunger; it's about fueling your mind for peak performance. The connection between diet and ADHD is strong, particularly in how blood sugar levels can sway your focus and mood. Imagine your brain as a high-performance engine that needs the right fuel to run smoothly. When your blood sugar dips, it can feel like hitting a wall, making concentration feel like an uphill battle. Conversely, a spike in blood sugar can lead to a whirlwind of energy followed by a crash, leaving you feeling drained and jittery. Maintaining stable blood sugar levels is crucial, as it helps sustain focus and a balanced mood throughout the day.

Nutrient deficiencies can also play a significant role in how you manage ADHD symptoms. When your body lacks essential nutrients, it's like trying to run a marathon without the proper shoes. For instance, a deficiency in omega-3 fatty acids can impair cognitive function, leaving you feeling foggy and distracted. These nutrients are vital for brain health, influencing everything from memory to the ability to concentrate. Ensuring you get an adequate intake of these essential nutrients can make a noticeable difference in how you feel and function daily.

Selecting ADHD-friendly foods is a step towards nourishing your brain effectively. Foods rich in omega-3 fatty acids, such as salmon or flaxseeds, are known to enhance cognitive performance, offering a natural boost to your mental clarity. Starting your day with a protein-rich breakfast can lay the groundwork for sustained energy and focus. Eggs, yogurt, or lean meats provide the protein your brain needs to stay sharp and attentive. Incorporating leafy greens and whole grains into your meals can further support your brain health. Spinach, kale, and whole-wheat bread are not only nutritious but also help maintain the steady energy levels your brain craves. These foods act like a steady hand on the steering wheel, guiding your brain through the twists and turns of the day with ease.

Meal planning and preparation might seem daunting in a busy schedule, but they're invaluable tools for maintaining a balanced diet. Prepping meals ahead of time can save you from the stress of last-minute decisions, ensuring you have nutritious options readily available. Consider setting aside time each week to chop vegetables or cook proteins that can be easily combined into meals. For those days when time is especially tight, meal kits or services can provide a convenient alternative without compromising on nutritional value. These kits often come with pre-portioned ingredients and easy-to-follow recipes, making it simple to whip up a healthy meal without the fuss. Planning grocery lists focused on whole foods can also streamline your shopping trips. By sticking to the perimeter of the grocery store, where most whole foods are found, you can fill your cart with fruits, vegetables, lean proteins, and whole grains that form the backbone of a brain-healthy diet.

Avoiding dietary pitfalls is just as crucial as selecting the right foods. Processed sugar is a common culprit that can wreak havoc on your focus and mood. While a sugary snack might offer a quick energy boost, it often leads to a sharp decline in concentration as your blood sugar levels plummet. Reducing caffeine consumption is another important step. While caffeine can temporarily enhance alertness, it may exacerbate anxiety and disrupt sleep, especially when combined with ADHD medications. Being mindful of potential food sensitivities can also make a difference. Certain foods, such as dairy or gluten, can trigger adverse reactions in some individuals, affecting their mood and focus. Paying attention to how your body responds to different foods can help you identify any sensitivities and adjust your diet accordingly.

EXERCISE AS A FOCUS ENHANCER

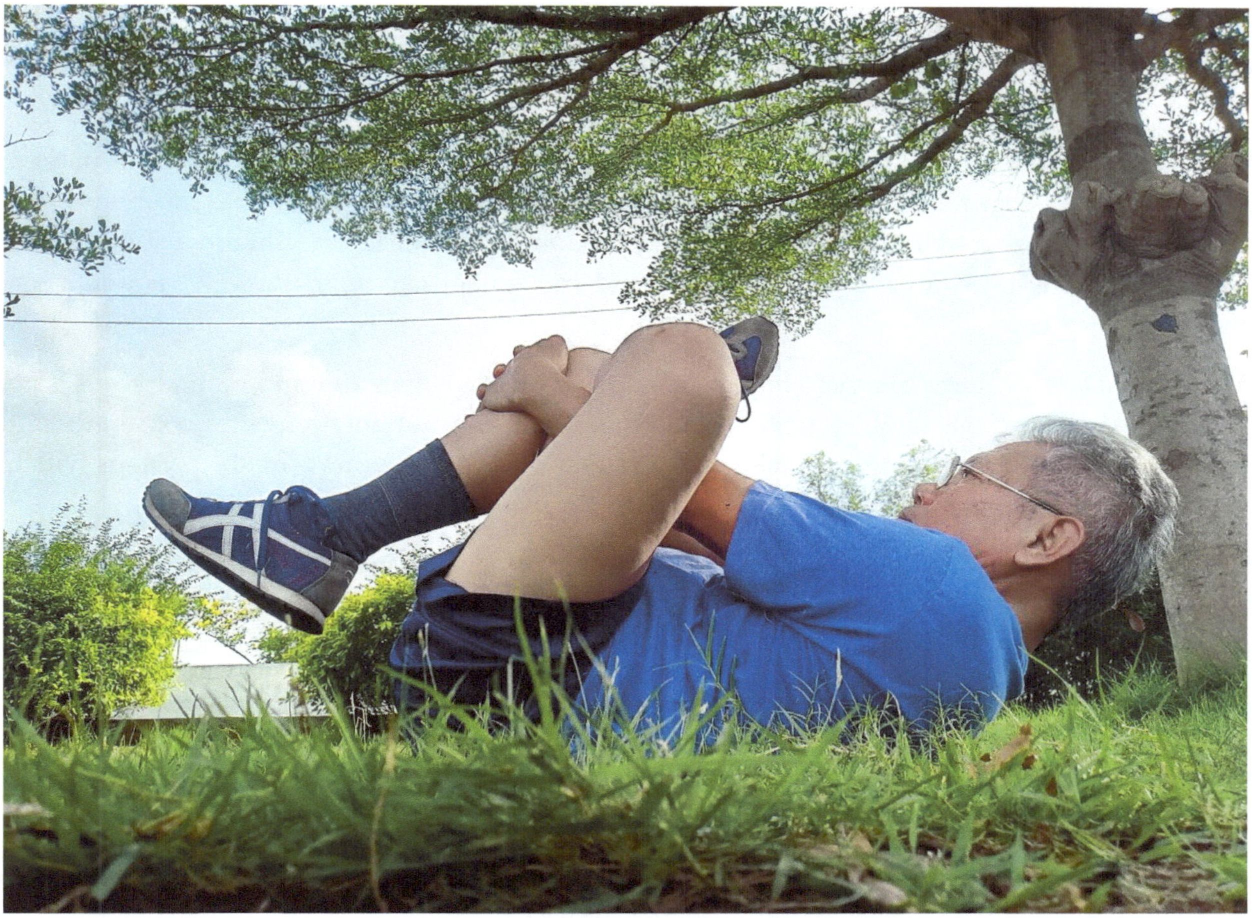

There are days when my mind feels like a crowded subway station during rush hour, with thoughts zooming past, seemingly without any order. It's on these days that I turn to exercise—not just as a way to keep fit, but as a tool to untangle the mess. Exercise gets my body moving, but more importantly, it gets my brain in gear. Physical activity triggers the release of neurotransmitters like dopamine, which play a crucial role in enhancing focus and mental clarity. This chemical boost is like hitting the refresh button on your brain, clearing the fog and sharpening your thoughts. Regular exercise doesn't just provide short-term clarity; it also promotes long-term brain health. By increasing blood flow and stimulating growth factors, exercise helps maintain brain plasticity, which is essential for learning and memory.

Finding the right form of exercise can be a game-changer, not only for your body but for your mind. It's about discovering what makes you feel alive, what gets your heart racing, and what brings a smile to your face. Group sports can be particularly beneficial, offering not just physical exertion but a chance for social interaction. Whether it's joining a local soccer team or hitting the basketball courts with friends, these activities can foster a sense of community and camaraderie.

If you're more inclined toward creative expression, dance classes might be your calling. Moving to the rhythm, letting your body flow with the music, can be both liberating and energizing. Or maybe the great outdoors is where you find peace. Activities like hiking or cycling allow you to connect with nature, offering a dual benefit of physical and mental rejuvenation. The key is to explore various forms and pinpoint what resonates with you the most.

Incorporating exercise into your daily routine might seem daunting, especially with a packed schedule. But it's entirely doable with a bit of creativity and planning. Walking meetings are a fantastic way to get moving without sacrificing productivity. Instead of sitting in a stuffy room, take your discussions outside. The fresh air and movement can spark new ideas and keep everyone engaged.

Active breaks at work are another simple yet effective method. Set a timer to remind yourself to stand up, stretch, or take a quick walk around the office. This not only refreshes your body but also recharges your focus. Setting achievable fitness goals is crucial. Start small—perhaps with a ten-minute workout each day—and gradually increase as you build stamina.

Fitness apps can provide motivation and a sense of accomplishment. They allow you to track your progress, set goals, and even challenge friends, turning exercise into a fun and rewarding part of your day.

Despite the benefits, sticking to an exercise routine can be challenging, especially during low-energy periods. Time management is often a hurdle, but it's important to remember that exercise doesn't have to be a huge time commitment. Short, high-intensity workouts can be just as effective as longer sessions. Identify pockets of time throughout your day where you can squeeze in a quick workout—during lunch breaks or even after dinner.

Maintaining motivation requires a bit of strategy. On days when energy is low, remind yourself of the benefits you've experienced in the past. Think about how good you feel after a workout, and let that motivate you. It can also help to mix things up to keep your routine exciting. Try a new class, switch up your playlist, or invite a friend to join you. Sometimes, just changing the scenery or routine can reignite your enthusiasm.

DIGITAL DETOX: RECONNECTING WITH THE PRESENT

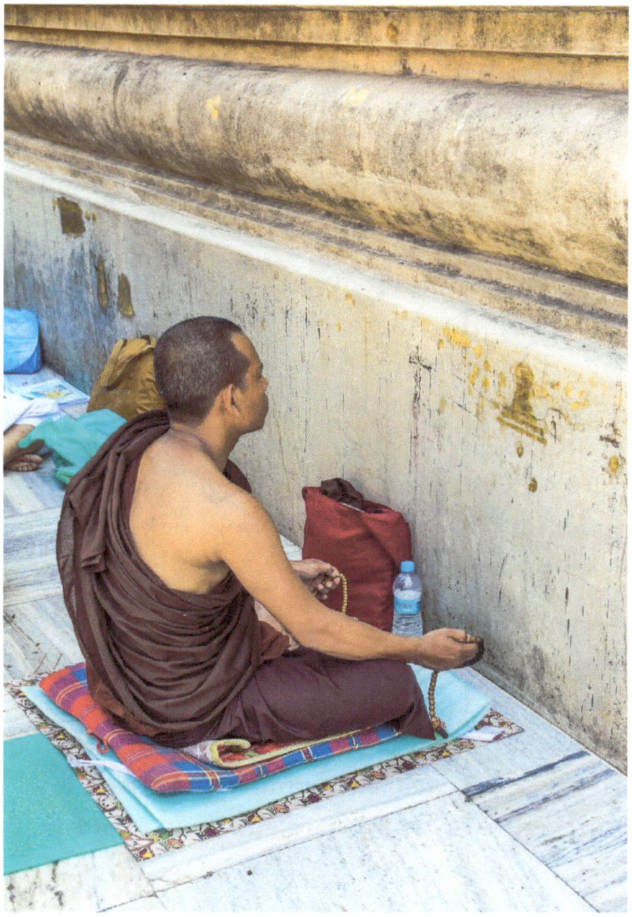

In today's world, our digital devices have become almost like extensions of ourselves. They're always within arm's reach, buzzing and beeping for our attention. While technology brings undeniable convenience, it also comes with its pitfalls, especially for those of us with ADHD. The constant influx of notifications can amplify the distractions we already grapple with, making it hard to focus on one task. Each alert pulls your attention away, leaving your mind scattered and your to-do list untouched. Over time, this digital overload can erode your ability to concentrate, leaving you more susceptible to the whims of the digital world. This distraction isn't just a minor inconvenience; it can significantly affect your productivity and mental health.

Moreover, the omnipresent glow of screens can wreak havoc with your sleep. The blue light emitted by phones, tablets, and computers can interfere with your body's natural sleep-wake cycle, making it harder to wind down and get a good night's rest. This disruption can be particularly troublesome for those with ADHD, as quality sleep is essential for managing symptoms like impulsivity and restlessness. Without it, you may find yourself in a cycle of fatigue and distraction, struggling to function at your best during the day. This vicious cycle can leave you feeling perpetually tired, exacerbating the very symptoms you're trying to manage.

Recognizing the signs that you might need a digital detox is the first step to reclaiming your mental clarity. If you find yourself constantly checking your devices out of habit rather than necessity, it might be time to step back. This compulsive behavior can create a sense of anxiety, making you feel tethered to your devices even during downtime. If the thought of being without your phone for an hour fills you with dread, or if you feel a pang of anxiety when you're disconnected, these are clear signals that a digital detox could be beneficial. Taking a break from screens can help reduce this anxiety, giving you the mental space to breathe and reconnect with the world around you.

Starting a digital detox doesn't have to be overwhelming. Begin by setting specific times for device-free periods. Maybe it's during meals, or perhaps you dedicate the first hour of your morning to being tech-free. These moments allow you to focus on being present, enjoying the company of loved ones, or simply savoring solitude. Creating tech-free zones in your home can further support this effort. Consider designating areas like the bedroom or dining room as screen-free spaces, encouraging more mindful engagement in these parts of your home. Engaging in offline activities such as reading, crafting, or even taking a walk can provide a refreshing change of pace, reminding you of the joys found beyond screens.

The benefits of reducing digital dependency are profound and far-reaching. By reducing screen time, you can enhance your mindfulness, becoming more attuned to the present moment. This heightened awareness can improve your focus, allowing you to engage more fully with the task at hand or the person in front of you. It also fosters improved interpersonal relationships and communication, as you're less distracted and more capable of giving others your undivided attention. This presence strengthens connections, making interactions more meaningful and enriching your social life.

As we wrap up this chapter, consider how these small changes can create ripples of positivity throughout your life. Reducing digital dependency isn't just about limiting screen time; it's about reclaiming your focus, nurturing relationships, and finding joy in the present. With these tools, you can foster a more balanced and fulfilling lifestyle. In the next chapter, we'll explore how to develop adaptive learning techniques that build on the foundation of self-care, allowing you to thrive in both personal and professional realms.

CHAPTER 8
DEVELOPING ADAPTIVE LEARNING TECHNIQUES

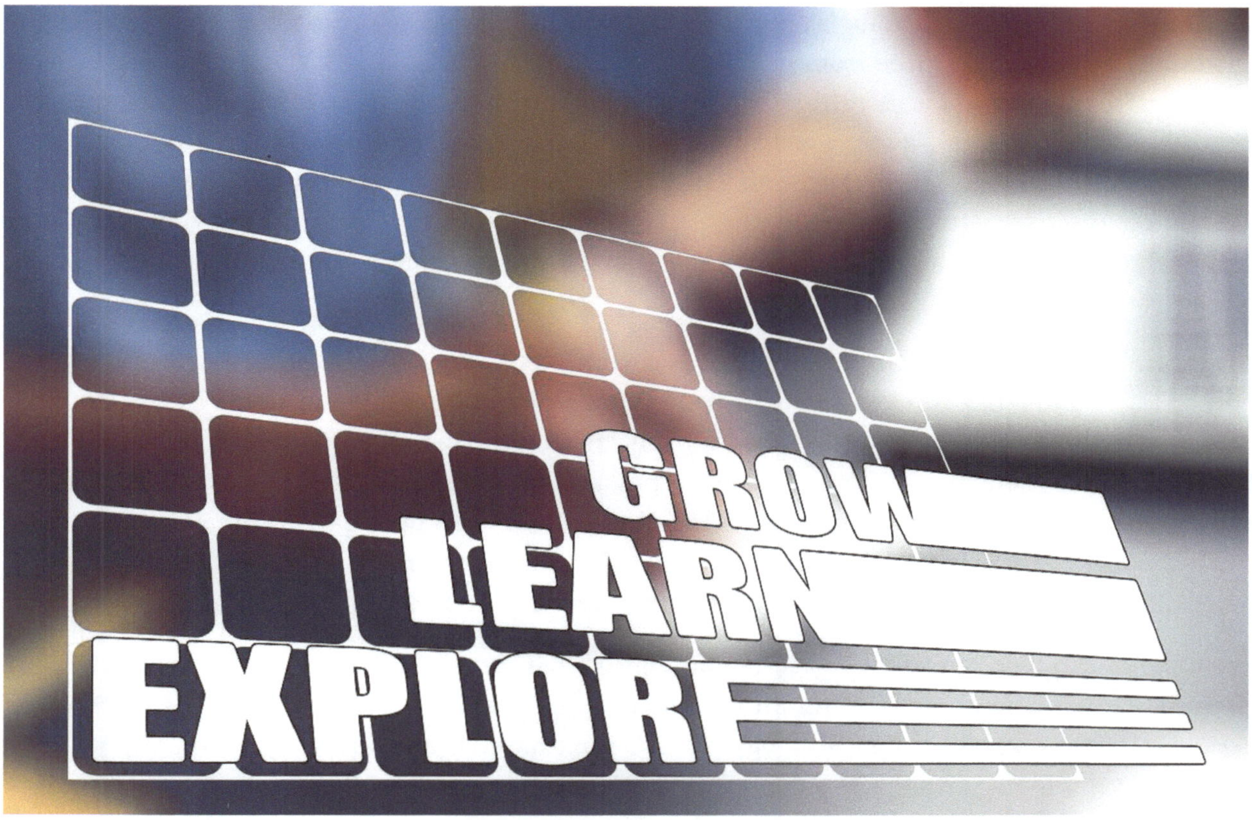

MY JOURNEY with ADHD has been like trying to tune into a distant radio station, where the signal is sometimes clear and other times filled with static. There was a time when I sat at my desk, a mountain of reading material in front of me, and found myself staring blankly at the pages. The words seemed to blur together as my mind wandered to a dozen different places. It was frustrating, to say the least, and I often wondered if I'd ever find a way to focus long enough to get through a chapter, let alone a book. Over time, I learned that ADHD doesn't mean you can't focus; it just means you focus differently. Understanding this has been a game-changer, and I've discovered some strategies that can help harness the unique way our brains work.

Attention variability is a hallmark of ADHD. Our ability to focus can be inconsistent, showing up in bursts that are as unpredictable as they are powerful. One minute, you're lost in thought, and the next, you're hyper-focused on a task that absorbs every ounce of your attention. This variability can be challenging, but it's also an opportunity to work with your brain, not against it. One key to managing this is identifying your peak focus times. Some people find they're more alert and engaged in the morning, while others hit their stride in the afternoon or evening. Recognizing these patterns can help you schedule tasks that require more concentration during your peak times, optimizing your natural rhythms.

Your environment plays a significant role in your ability to focus. A cluttered or noisy space can be a minefield of distractions, while a well-organized environment can enhance your attention. Creating a distraction-free zone is crucial for those of us with ADHD. Start by setting up a dedicated study space that is free from clutter and interruptions. This space should be your sanctuary, a place where you can retreat to focus without the usual distractions. Noise-canceling headphones can be a lifesaver, especially if you live in a bustling household or work in a busy office. They help block out background noise, allowing you to concentrate on the task at hand. Removing digital distractions is another vital step. Website blockers can prevent you from wandering onto social media or other time-wasting sites, keeping your focus where it needs to be.

Incorporating focus-enhancing techniques into your study sessions can make a world of difference. Fidget tools, like stress balls or fidget spinners, can help maintain focus by giving your hands something to do while your mind concentrates on the task. These tools offer a subtle way to channel excess energy, making it easier to pay attention. Regular physical movement breaks are also essential. Sitting still for long periods can be tough, so taking short breaks to stretch or walk around can refresh your mind and improve concentration. These breaks act as a mental reset, allowing you to return to your work with renewed focus and energy.

Technology can be a powerful ally in managing focus. There are countless apps designed to aid time management and provide reminders. Apps like Forest or Focus@Will can help structure your time and keep distractions at bay. Forest, for example, encourages you to stay off your phone by growing a virtual tree as you focus, offering a visual representation of your progress. Digital timers can also be incredibly useful, helping you break your work into manageable chunks. By setting a timer for specific intervals, you create a sense of urgency and focus, making it easier to tackle tasks without getting overwhelmed.

Interactive Element: Peak Focus Time Journal

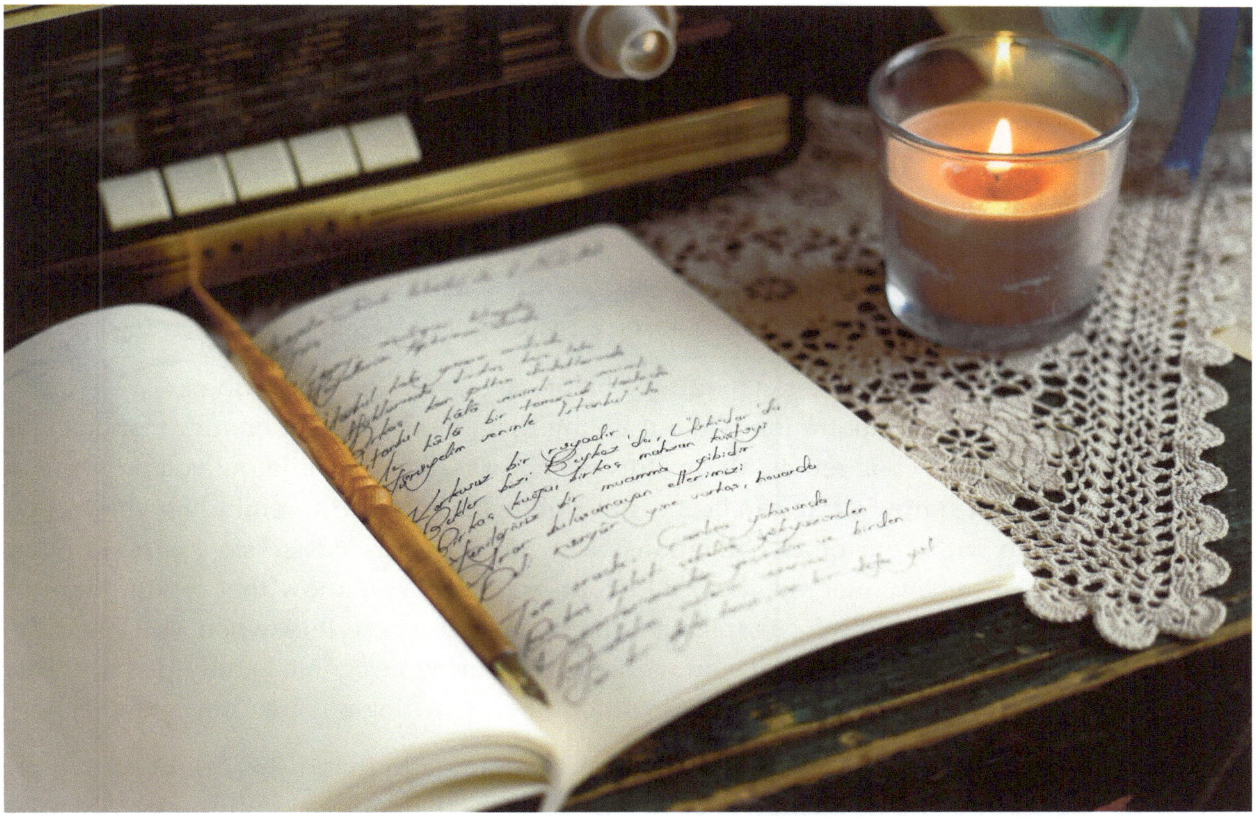

To better understand your attention patterns, try keeping a journal to track your peak focus times. Note the times of day when you feel most alert and engaged, as well as the times when concentration seems to slip away. Reflect on any environmental factors that might influence your focus, such as noise levels or clutter. Use this information to adjust your schedule, plan demanding tasks during your peak times, and use less focused periods for routine or less important activities. This exercise can help you align your work with your natural rhythms, enhancing productivity and reducing frustration.

HARNESSING HYPERFOCUS FOR LEARNING

Hyperfocus is one of those double-edged swords in the world of ADHD. It's like having a superpower that lets you zero in on a task with laser-like precision. When you're in a state of hyperfocus, everything else seems to fade away, and you're able to dive into deep learning with incredible intensity. This can lead to moments of brilliance where you absorb information like a sponge, understanding complexities that usually seem out of reach. But, as with any superpower, there are drawbacks. Hyperfocus can sometimes cause you to neglect other responsibilities or lose track of time entirely, leaving you scrambling to catch up on forgotten tasks.

Recognizing both the benefits and pitfalls of hyperfocus is key to using it effectively in your learning process.

Identifying what triggers your hyperfocus is like finding the key to a treasure chest. Think back to times when you became so engrossed in an activity that hours flew by without notice. What were you doing? These moments often hold clues to the subjects or activities that naturally engage your hyperfocus. Reflect on these experiences to pinpoint your triggers. Maybe it's a particular topic you're passionate about or a specific type of challenge that grabs your attention. To refine this understanding, experiment with diverse topics and activities. Try new things and observe how your focus responds. You might discover that certain subjects ignite your curiosity and draw you into a hyper-focused state, offering a roadmap for directing your learning efforts.

Balancing hyperfocus with other tasks requires a bit of strategy. It's about finding a way to enjoy those periods of intense concentration without letting them derail the rest of your responsibilities. One effective approach is setting alarms to signal breaks. When you know you're prone to losing track of time, a simple alarm can be a gentle nudge back to reality, reminding you to step away and check in with your other obligations. Scheduling hyperfocus sessions around other commitments can also help integrate them into your routine. If you know that certain times of day tend to trigger your hyperfocus, plan to engage in those activities when you have the freedom to fully immerse yourself—like on weekends or during designated study periods. This way, you can enjoy the benefits of hyperfocus without it encroaching on other important tasks.

Maximizing your learning during hyperfocus means tapping into that deep well of concentration for educational gain. One method is to engage in deep-dive projects with research components. Choose a topic that piques your interest and allows you to explore it thoroughly. This approach not only satisfies your curiosity but also builds your knowledge base in a meaningful way. Intensive study sessions with specific objectives can also be highly effective during hyperfocus. Set clear goals for what you want to achieve in each session, whether it's mastering a new concept or completing a section of a project. Having these concrete objectives gives your hyperfocus direction and purpose, enabling you to channel your attention productively.

Hyperfocus can be a formidable ally in your learning toolkit. By understanding what triggers this state and learning to balance it with your other responsibilities, you can harness its power to enhance your educational experiences. Embrace those moments of intense concentration, and let them guide you to deeper understanding and insight.

CREATIVE NOTE-TAKING TECHNIQUES

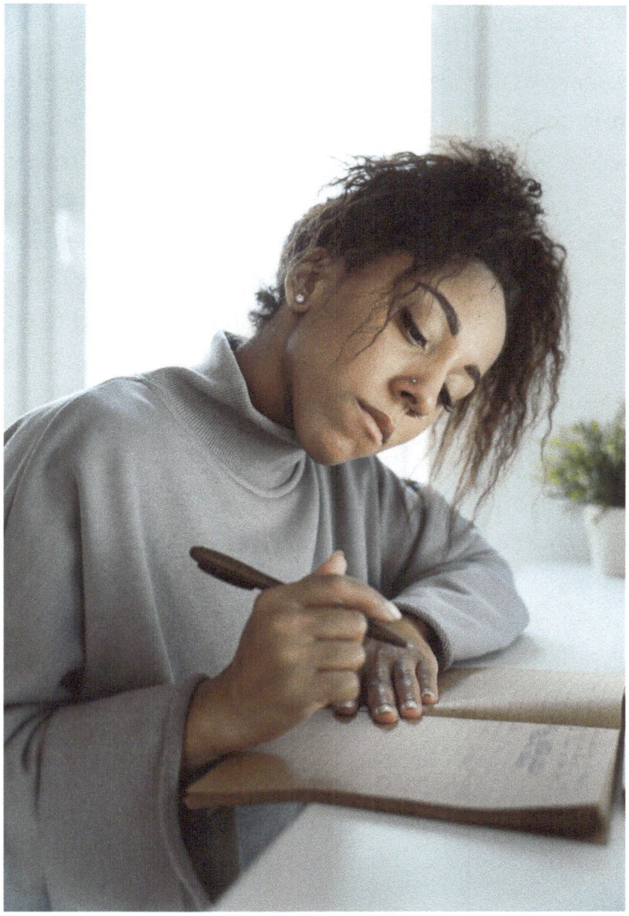

Note-taking has always felt like a lifeline for me, especially when navigating the whirlwind of thoughts that come with ADHD. It's not just about jotting down what's important; it's about creating a map that guides you through the maze of information. Creative note-taking can make all the difference in how we retain and understand what we learn. For visual learners, the graphic representation of ideas can be transformative. Imagine turning a dense block of text into a colorful diagram or sketch that captures the essence of the material. This approach doesn't just simplify complex information; it brings it to life, allowing you to see connections and patterns that might otherwise be obscured.

There are endless ways to take notes, and finding the right style can turn a chore into an engaging task. Mind mapping is one of my favorites. It organizes information visually, with a central idea branching out into related topics. This method mirrors the way our brains naturally process information, making it easier to recall later. Bullet journaling is another great option, offering a structured way to organize notes while allowing for flexibility. It combines the precision of lists with the freedom to add symbols and colors, creating a personalized system that evolves with your needs. Then there's sketch-noting, which combines visuals and text in a dynamic way. By drawing symbols, doodles, and diagrams alongside your notes, you tap into both hemispheres of your brain, enhancing your understanding and retention. These methods cater to different learning preferences, offering a toolkit that can be customized to suit you.

Personalizing your notes can make them more engaging and memorable. Color coding is a simple yet powerful technique. By assigning different colors to categories or themes, you create a visual cue that helps you organize and retrieve information. Imagine looking at a page of notes and instantly seeing the connections between related topics because they share the same color. Adding personal anecdotes or examples is another way to enrich your notes. When you tie new information to personal experiences, it becomes more relatable and easier to remember. Think of it as creating a story where you're the main character, and the concepts you're learning are part of your narrative. This personalization not only makes note-taking more enjoyable but also deepens your connection to the material.

In today's digital age, we have access to tools that can elevate our note-taking to new heights. Apps like Trello and OneNote offer platforms for organizing and storing notes in a way that suits your workflow. Trello's card system is perfect for tracking tasks and ideas, while OneNote's digital notebooks allow for endless customization. Both apps offer features like tagging and search functions, making it easy to find and revisit past notes. For those who prefer a tactile approach, digital tablets with stylus capabilities offer a bridge between traditional and digital note-taking. With a digital tablet, you can sketch, write, and annotate with ease, and the ability to sync your notes across devices ensures they're always within reach. These tools open up a world of possibilities, allowing you to experiment and find what works best for you.

VISUAL ELEMENT: NOTE-TAKING STYLES INFOGRAPHIC

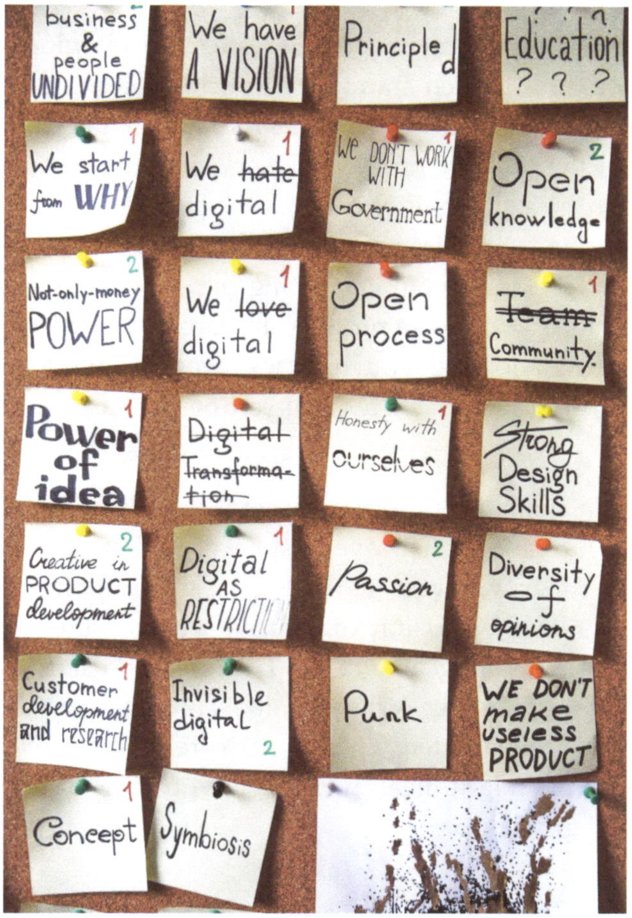

Consider creating an infographic that showcases different note-taking styles, like mind mapping, bullet journaling, and sketch-noting. Include visuals and brief descriptions of each method, highlighting their unique benefits. This visual element can serve as a quick reference guide, helping you choose the style that resonates with your learning preferences. Use it to inspire your note-taking practice and remind yourself of the creative possibilities that await.

Setting Learning Goals That Stick

Setting goals can sometimes feel like staring at a blank canvas, unsure of where to begin. But much like painting, once you make that first brushstroke, the rest starts to take shape. In learning, setting clear goals acts as a guiding light, providing direction and motivation. Without them, it's easy to drift aimlessly, losing focus and momentum. Specific and measurable goals are crucial because they give you something tangible to aim for. Instead of saying, "I want to get better at math," a more effective goal would be, "I will practice algebra for 30 minutes a day, five days a week." This kind of clarity not only makes your objectives more attainable but also aligns them with your interests and strengths, ensuring that your efforts are both meaningful and rewarding.

There are several frameworks you can use to set effective learning goals. One of the most popular is the SMART method, which stands for Specific, Measurable, Achievable, Relevant, and Time-bound. This approach breaks down goals into actionable steps, providing a clear path to follow. Each element of the SMART framework serves a purpose: specificity sharpens focus, measurability tracks progress, achievability ensures the goal is within reach, relevance ties it to personal interests, and setting a time frame creates urgency. Another useful model is OKRs, or Objectives and Key Results. OKRs encourage setting big, ambitious objectives and then identifying measurable key results that indicate progress toward those objectives. This method fosters both vision and practicality, allowing you to track progress while remaining flexible. Both frameworks offer a structured approach to goal-setting that can significantly enhance your learning journey.

The path to achieving your goals isn't always smooth. Life throws curveballs, and it's easy to stumble along the way. Motivation can waver, especially when facing setbacks. During these times, it's essential to remember why you set the goal in the first place. Reconnecting with your initial motivation can reignite the passion that drove you to start. Consider breaking down larger goals into smaller, more manageable tasks. This creates a series of quick wins that build confidence and keep momentum going. Adjusting goals is okay, too. Circumstances change, and sometimes, goals need to be reevaluated. The key is to remain flexible without losing sight of the overarching objective. This might mean revising time frames or altering the steps you need to take, but it doesn't mean giving up.

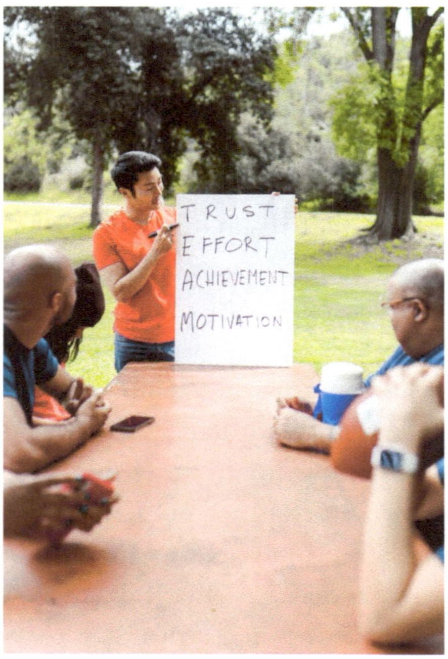

Celebrating milestones and successes is crucial for sustaining motivation. Each achievement, no matter how small, is a testament to your progress and effort. Create a reward system that acknowledges these accomplishments. Rewards don't have to be extravagant; they can be as simple as taking a break to watch your favorite show or treating yourself to a favorite snack. The important thing is to acknowledge your hard work in a way that feels meaningful to you. Reflecting on your progress through a learning journal can also be a valuable exercise. By regularly documenting your achievements and challenges, you gain insights into your learning process and growth. This practice not only reinforces your successes but also helps you identify areas for improvement, creating a continuous cycle of learning and development.

Setting goals transcends mere achievement; they are milestones on your journey of personal and intellectual growth. Establishing clear, attainable objectives crafts a roadmap that not only guides your learning journey but also fosters resilience and motivates you to stretch your boundaries. The fulfillment derived from accomplishing these goals propels you toward new horizons of discovery, bolstering your confidence and enriching your appreciation for the learning process. This chapter underscores the vital role of clear, structured, and celebratory goal-setting in fostering significant personal development. Moving forward, we will explore the art of decision-making, focusing on how to navigate choices confidently and adapt to change gracefully.

CHAPTER 9
DECISION-MAKING WITH CONFIDENCE

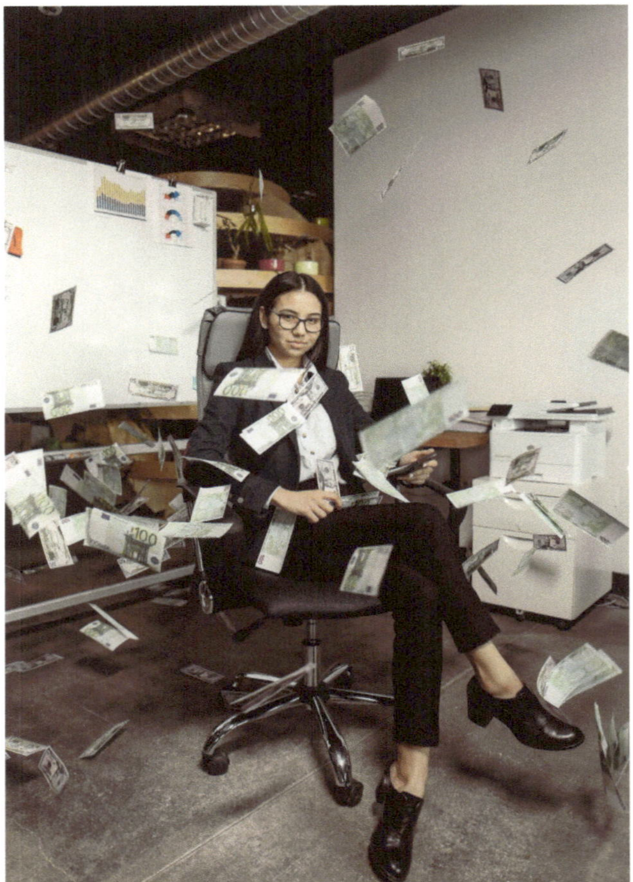

THE OTHER DAY, I found myself standing in the cereal aisle of the grocery store, paralyzed by the sheer number of choices. I'm often paralyzed by the amount of decisions I have to make.

It was just cereal, but my mind was buzzing with indecision. This moment, trivial as it may seem, encapsulates a common challenge for many of us with ADHD: decision-making fatigue. It's not just about choosing between cereals; it's about the constant stream of decisions that bombard us throughout the day. From what to have for breakfast to which project to tackle first, each choice chips away at our mental energy, leaving us exhausted and sometimes even questioning our decisions. Yet, in a world that demands quick thinking, the ability to make decisions efficiently is invaluable, especially in fast-paced work environments where opportunities can vanish as quickly as they appear.

In these settings, the need for rapid decision-making becomes clear. It's not just about keeping up with the speed of business but also about reducing decision fatigue, a phenomenon in which the quality of decisions deteriorates after a long session. When every choice feels monumental, it can lead to analysis paralysis, where too many options freeze us in place. By honing the skill of quick decision-making, you can preserve your mental resources for when they're truly needed, ensuring that each decision is made with clarity and purpose.

One technique that has revolutionized my approach to decision-making is the two-minute rule. It's simple: if a decision or task can be completed in two minutes or less, do it immediately. This rule helps cut through the noise of indecision, allowing you to clear minor tasks and decisions off your plate swiftly. By adopting this approach, you free up mental space for more significant decisions, reducing the overall cognitive load.

In conjunction with this, blending intuition with logical reasoning can be powerful. People with ADHD often possess a sharp, intuitive sense that can guide them in making effective decisions quickly. By trusting this intuition while applying a logical framework, you can navigate decisions with confidence, even when time is limited.

Practical tools and techniques can be invaluable to further streamline the decision-making process. Decision trees provide a visual representation of choices and potential outcomes, making complex decisions more manageable by breaking them down into smaller, more digestible parts. Similarly, creating a pros and cons list can offer clarity, allowing you to weigh options quickly and objectively. Digital tools, such as decision-making apps, can also support this process by organizing options and outcomes, ensuring that you have all the necessary information at your fingertips. These tools not only speed up decision-making but also enhance accuracy, helping you make informed choices that align with your goals.

Despite these strategies, the fear of making mistakes often looms large, casting a shadow over decision-making processes. This fear, while understandable, can be paralyzing, preventing you from moving forward and seizing opportunities. However, mistakes are not the end of the world; they're stepping stones to growth and learning. By viewing mistakes as valuable learning opportunities, you can reframe your perspective, transforming fear into motivation. Each mistake offers insights into what didn't work and why, providing the chance to refine your approach and improve future decisions.

To mitigate the impact of potential mistakes, consider implementing strategies that minimize their consequences. This might involve planning for contingencies or seeking feedback from trusted colleagues or mentors before committing to a decision. By building a support system around your decision-making process, you create a safety net that allows you to take calculated risks without fear of catastrophic failure. This approach not only bolsters your confidence but also fosters a culture of resilience, where you can adapt and thrive in the face of uncertainty.

Interactive Element: Decision-Making Reflection Exercise

Take a moment to reflect on a recent decision that left you feeling uncertain or anxious. Consider the following prompts: What factors influenced your decision? How did you weigh the options? What was the outcome, and what did you learn from it? Write down your reflections in a journal, noting any patterns or insights that emerge. This exercise can help you identify strengths and areas for growth in your decision-making process, empowering you to make more confident and informed choices in the future.

NAVIGATING MAJOR LIFE CHOICES

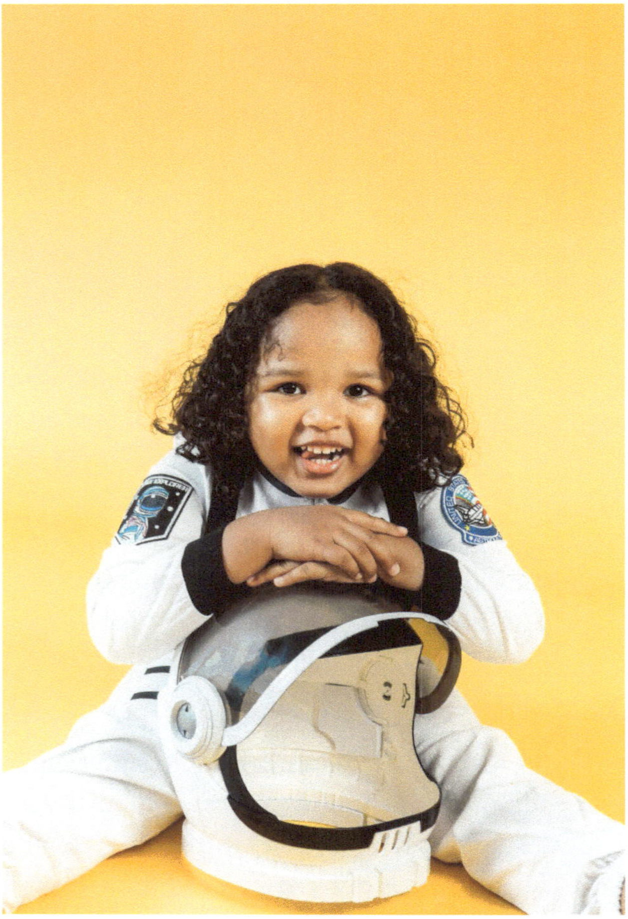

When it comes to making significant life decisions, the stakes feel high. These aren't just run-of-the-mill choices like what to wear or eat; these decisions can alter the course of your life. Think about career changes or relocations. Deciding to switch careers can feel like standing at the edge of a cliff, looking out at a vast yet unknown landscape. There's excitement, sure, but also a hefty dose of fear. What if the new job doesn't work out? What if moving to a new city leaves you feeling isolated? These choices often come with a domino effect, impacting your social life, financial stability, and overall happiness. Then, there are decisions about significant relationships—whether to commit long-term or step away. The emotional weight of these choices can be daunting, yet they are necessary for personal growth and fulfillment.

Structured frameworks can be a lifesaver for tackling such complex decisions. One approach is the DECIDE model, which breaks down the process into manageable steps. Start by defining the problem clearly, then explore your options. Consider the pros and cons, identify the best choice, develop a plan, and finally, evaluate the outcome. This model provides a roadmap that helps prevent feeling overwhelmed by the enormity of the decision. Another useful tool is the SWOT analysis, which examines strengths, weaknesses, opportunities, and threats related to your decision. By laying everything out, you gain a clearer picture of the potential paths and their implications. These frameworks offer structure and clarity, making it easier to approach decisions with confidence.

Gathering relevant information is crucial in making informed choices. It's like assembling the pieces of a puzzle before you start. Consulting experts or mentors can provide insights you might not have considered. Their experience offers a perspective that can illuminate blind spots you might have overlooked. Conducting scenario analysis is another powerful technique. Imagine the different outcomes each decision might lead to, considering the best and worst-case scenarios. This helps you prepare for various eventualities, reducing the uncertainty that often clouds major decisions. Reviewing past experiences is equally valuable. Look back at similar decisions you've made before—what worked, what didn't, and what lessons did you learn? These reflections guide you away from past mistakes and toward more informed choices.

Balancing emotion and logic is perhaps one of the most challenging aspects of decision-making. It's easy to get swept away by emotions, whether they're fueled by fear, excitement, or pressure from others. However, integrating emotional and rational considerations leads to more grounded decisions. Techniques for emotional regulation can help maintain this balance. Practice mindfulness to stay present and avoid being hijacked by emotion. It's about pausing, taking a breath, and allowing yourself to find a calm space before reacting. Ensure that your decisions align with your core values and long-term goals. Ask yourself if the choice supports your vision for your life, not just in the present moment but also in the future. This alignment acts as a compass, guiding you through the noise and keeping you true to yourself.

ANALYZING RISK VS. REWARD

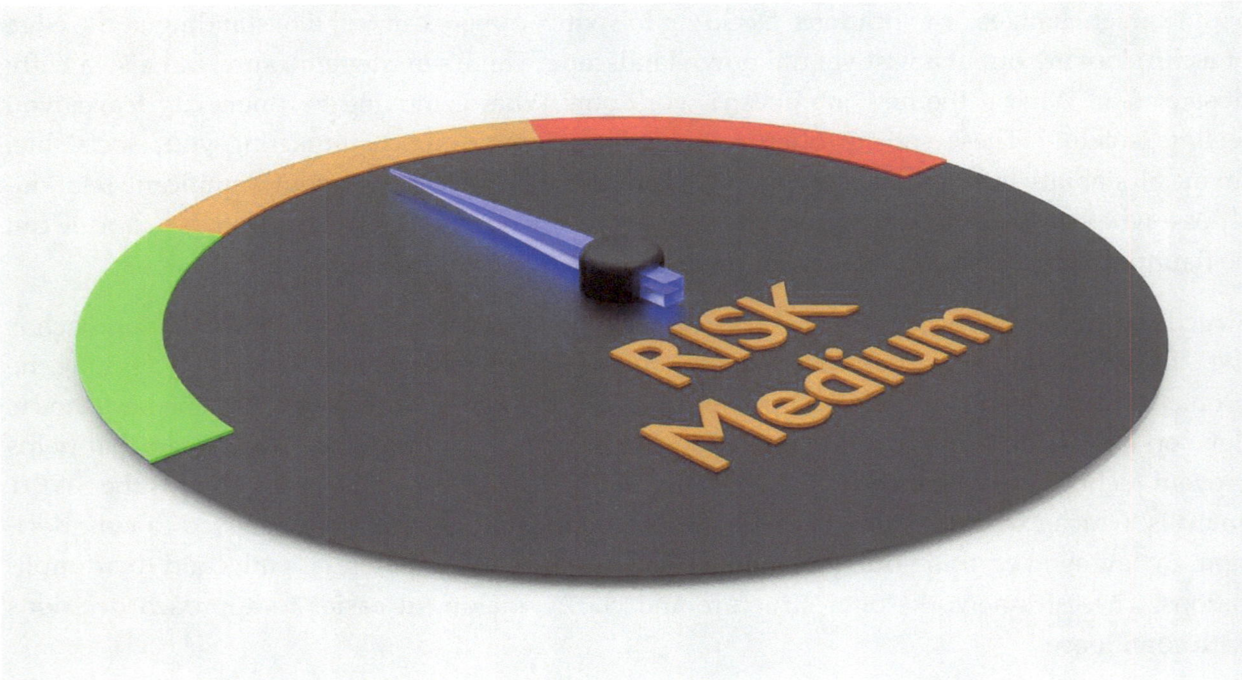

Risk and reward are two sides of the same coin, intricately linked in every decision we make. When considering a decision, it's crucial to weigh the potential gains against the possible losses. Imagine you're contemplating investing in a new business venture. The allure of high returns might be tempting, but it's essential to balance this with the risk of losing your initial investment. Understanding this dynamic involves not just a gut feeling but a careful calculation of what you're willing to risk to achieve your desired outcome. This is where identifying acceptable levels of risk comes into play. It's about knowing your limits and understanding how much you're comfortable putting on the line. This awareness helps you make choices that align with your financial goals and personal tolerance for uncertainty.

Practical tools and methods can be your best allies when assessing risks effectively. One such tool is the risk matrix, which offers a clear visual representation of risk levels by plotting the likelihood of an event against its potential impact. This matrix helps you prioritize risks, focusing on those that are both likely to occur and carry significant consequences. It simplifies complex scenarios by categorizing risks into manageable sections, enabling you to see where your attention is most needed. Another valuable method is cost-benefit analysis, which evaluates the trade-offs of a decision by comparing its expected benefits and associated costs. This approach allows you to quantify the value of a decision, providing a clear picture of whether the potential reward justifies the risk involved. Probability assessments also play a crucial role in estimating the likelihood of various outcomes. By analyzing data and trends, you can make informed predictions about future events, enhancing your ability to manage risks proactively.

Once you've identified the risks, it's time to strategize on how to mitigate them. Diversification is a tried-and-true strategy, particularly in financial decisions. By spreading investments across different assets, you reduce the impact of a poor-performing investment on your overall portfolio. It's the classic "don't put all your eggs in one basket" approach, ensuring that a single setback doesn't derail your entire financial plan. Contingency planning is another powerful tool in your risk management arsenal. It involves preparing for unexpected outcomes by having backup plans in place. This could mean setting aside emergency funds or developing alternative strategies to pivot when things don't go as planned. By anticipating potential challenges and having solutions ready, you can navigate setbacks with greater confidence and ease.

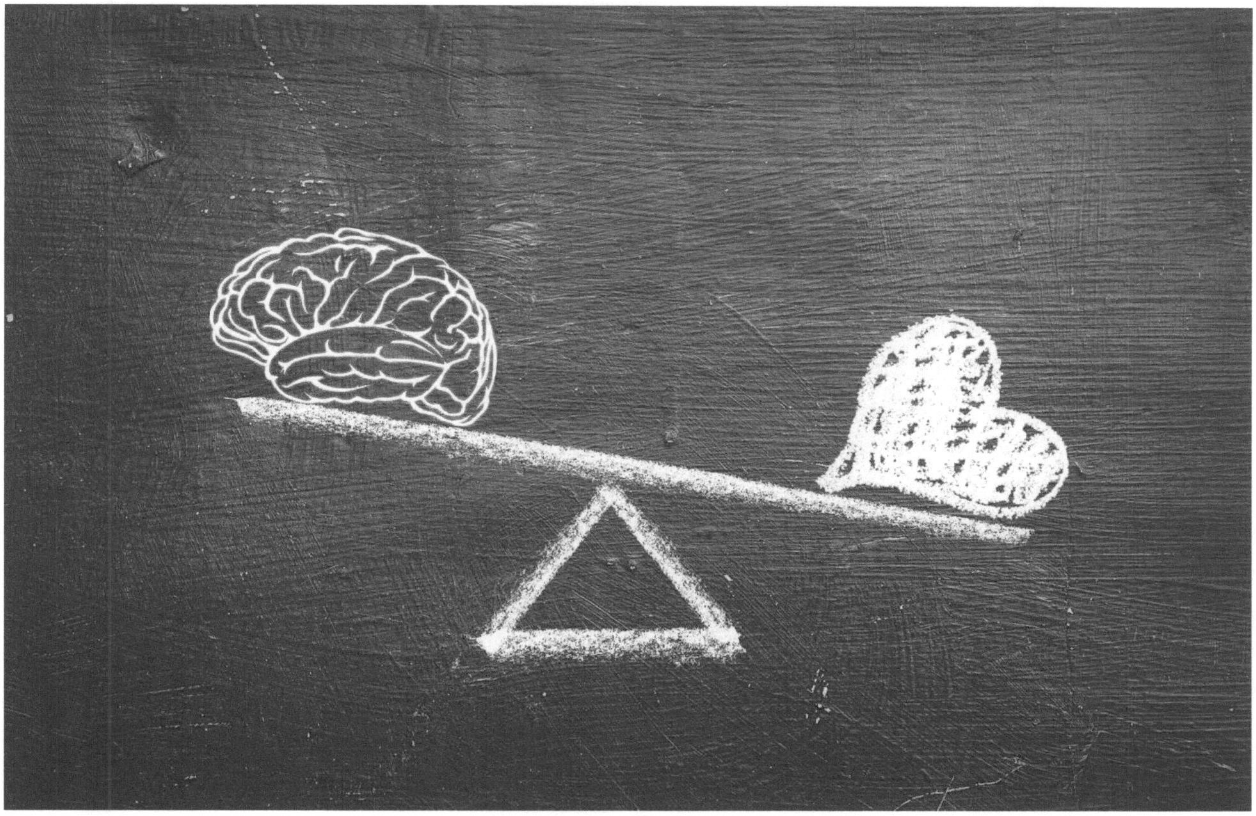

Examining real-life examples of successful risk management can offer valuable insights into effective strategies. Consider the world of entrepreneurial ventures, where risk is a constant companion. Entrepreneurs often face high stakes, but those who succeed typically do so by embracing calculated risks. They analyze potential opportunities, prepare for obstacles, and adapt their strategies as needed. Take, for example, the story of a tech startup that faced financial struggles but managed to pivot its business model successfully. By re-evaluating its risks and adjusting its approach, the company turned its fortunes around, eventually becoming a market leader. Similarly, historical decisions in business or public policy provide lessons in risk management. Governments and organizations often make decisions that carry significant risks, such as implementing new policies or entering foreign markets. By studying these cases, you can learn how others have balanced risk and reward, applying these lessons to your own decision-making process.

EMBRACING CHANGE: TRANSITIONING SMOOTHLY

Change is this strange thing that can both excite and terrify us. On one hand, it promises new beginnings and opportunities; on the other, it can throw us into chaos. Psychologically, change can stir up a whole mix of emotions—fear, anxiety, and even resistance. It's natural to feel a bit rattled when faced with the unknown. Resistance often stems from our brain's desire to keep us safe in familiar territory, where the risks are minimal. But what happens when staying put isn't an option? That's when the stress creeps in. Understanding this resistance is the first step in managing it. It's okay to feel uneasy; it's a sign you're stepping out of your comfort zone. This is where coping mechanisms come into play. Simple practices like mindfulness or deep breathing can help ground you. Even talking it out with a friend or therapist can work wonders, giving you a space to process your feelings without judgment.

Preparing for change is a bit like packing for a trip. You want to make sure you have everything you need, but you also don't want to carry unnecessary baggage. Establishing a support network is crucial. Surround yourself with people who understand and support the changes you're making. They can offer guidance, share their experiences, and provide a listening ear when things get tough. Setting realistic expectations and timelines is equally important. It's easy to get caught up in the excitement of change and set goals that are too ambitious. Break down your transition into manageable steps, and give yourself plenty of time to adjust. Remember, change doesn't happen overnight, and that's perfectly alright. Taking it one day at a time can help ease the pressure and make the process more enjoyable.

Adapting to new circumstances requires a mindset that's open and willing to embrace the unknown. Flexibility is your greatest ally here. It's about being open to new possibilities and not being too rigid in your plans. Sometimes, the best opportunities come from unexpected places. Developing new routines is another way to create stability amidst change. Routines provide a sense of normalcy and can help anchor you when everything else feels up in the air. They don't have to be elaborate—just simple daily practices that ground you. And let's not forget about seeking growth opportunities in the midst of change. Every transition is an opportunity to learn something new about yourself or the world around you. Whether it's picking up a new skill, meeting new people, or exploring new interests, embracing change can lead to personal growth in ways you might not have imagined.

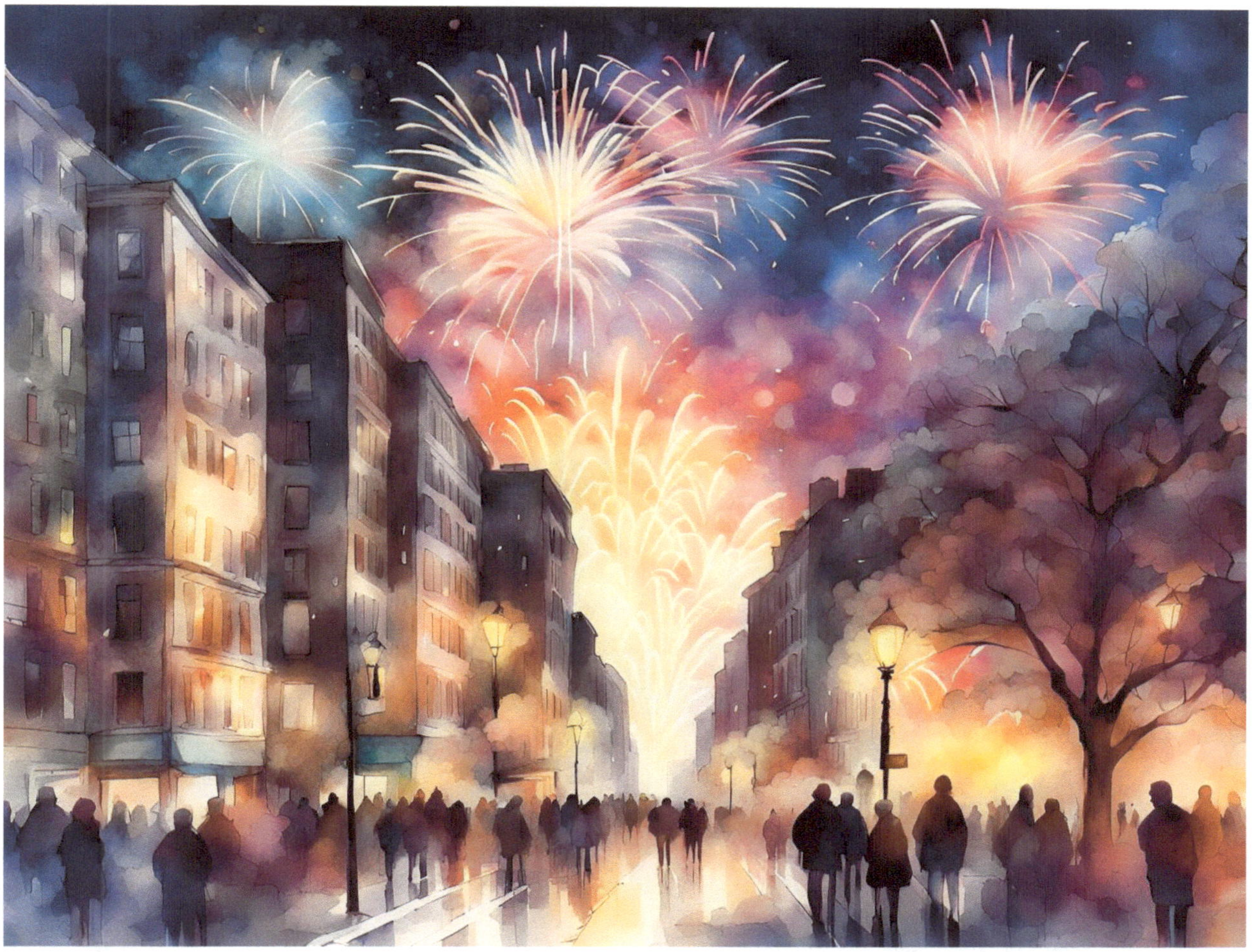

Celebrating progress during transitions is something we often overlook. We're so focused on the end goal that we forget to acknowledge the small victories along the way. Take time to reflect on your personal growth and achievements, no matter how minor they may seem. Each step forward is progress, and it deserves recognition. Consider rewarding yourself when you reach certain milestones. It could be something as simple as treating yourself to a nice meal or taking a day off to relax. These rewards serve as reminders of how far you've come and motivate you to keep pushing forward.

As we wrap up this chapter on embracing change, remember that transitions are not just about getting from point A to point B. They're about the journey—each step, each learning, and each moment of growth. In the next chapter, we'll explore how creativity and innovation can be harnessed to further enhance your ADHD potential, opening doors to new possibilities and achievements.

CHAPTER 10
EMBRACING CHANGE AND OVERCOMING CHALLENGES

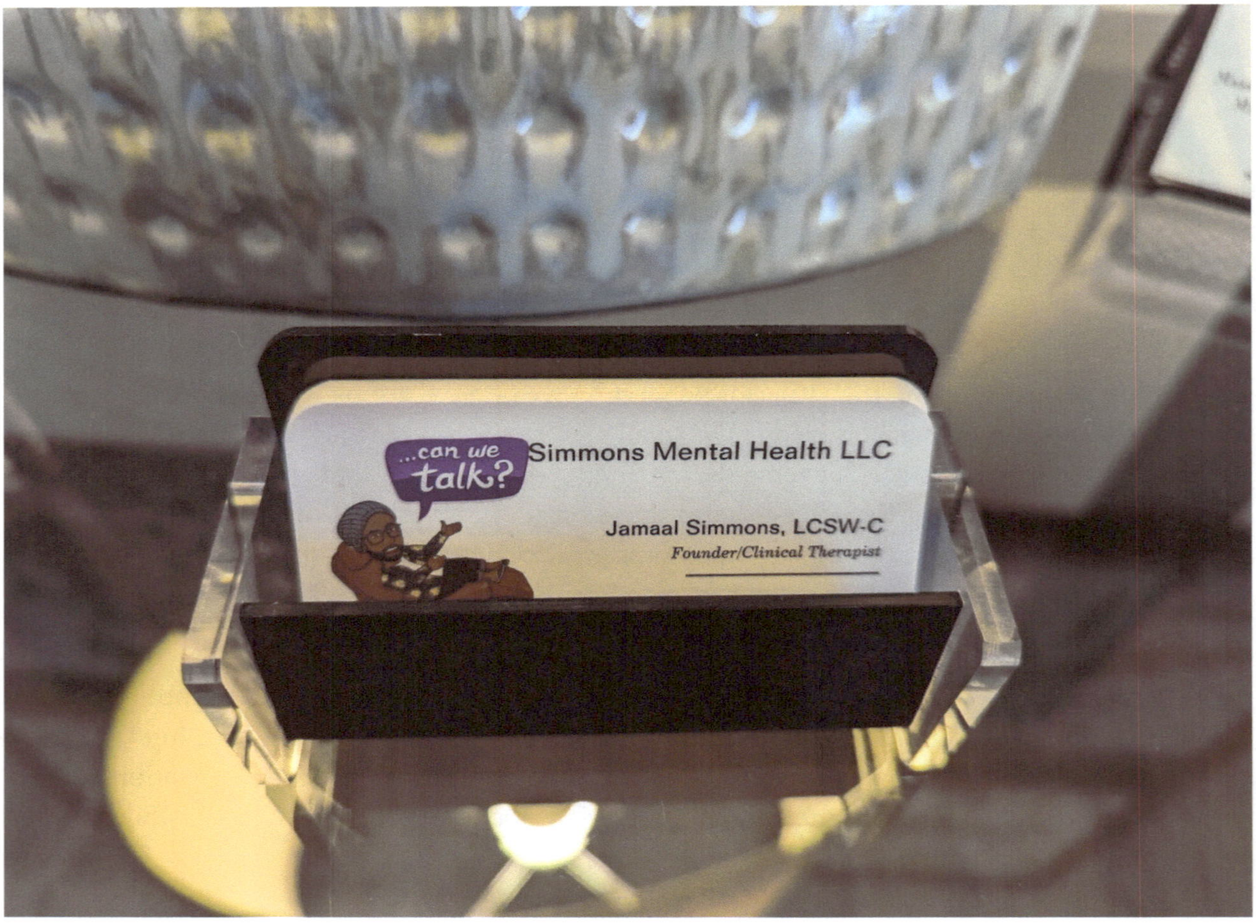

My "not boring" business card for Simmons Mental Health LLC

LIFE OFTEN FEELS like a series of unexpected, knife-twisting plot twists, doesn't it? Just when you think you've got everything figured out, the universe throws a curveball your way. I remember a time when I was sure I was on the right track. I had a plan, a vision, and a checklist. Yet, I found myself staring at a depressing closed door that I hadn't anticipated—a job opportunity dissolved unexpectedly, leaving me standing there, confused and a bit defeated. It was in that moment of uncertainty that I stumbled upon the idea of mindset, specifically the concept of a growth mindset. It was like finding a new pair of glasses that made everything clearer, turning what felt like an insurmountable obstacle into a stepping stone for growth.

BUILDING A GROWTH MINDSET

The idea of a growth mindset, introduced by psychologist Carol Dweck, is a game-changer—especially for those of us navigating the ADHD landscape. It's all about the belief that our abilities, intelligence, and talents aren't fixed traits. Instead, they can develop over time through dedication, effort, and learning. Contrast this with a fixed mindset, where abilities are seen as static, leading to a fear of failure and a tendency to shy away from challenges. For adults with ADHD, this fixed mindset can be a real barrier, often reinforced by years of negative self-talk and perceived limitations.

Embracing a growth mindset means seeing challenges not as threats but as opportunities to learn and grow. It encourages us to persist in the face of setbacks, understanding that struggle is part of the improvement process. This perspective allows us to approach life's hurdles with curiosity and resilience, rather than avoidance and anxiety. For those with ADHD, adopting a growth mindset can increase motivation and engagement, both personally and professionally. It creates a framework where setbacks are not failures but rather stepping stones to greater understanding and success.

Cultivating a growth mindset involves a conscious shift in how we interpret challenges. Instead of viewing obstacles as roadblocks, try to see them as puzzles waiting to be solved. Reframing challenges in this way can transform your approach to problem-solving.

Embrace self-reflection and seek feedback from others. This practice helps you see different perspectives and find areas for improvement. Focus on setting learning goals rather than performance goals. Learning goals emphasize the process and encourage a love for discovery, while performance goals often focus solely on outcomes, which can be discouraging if not immediately achieved.

Incorporating a growth mindset into daily life can be as simple as keeping a journal. Reflect on your experiences each day, noting what you learned from both successes and failures. Celebrate effort and progress, not just the end results. This practice reinforces that growth happens over time and through effort, not overnight. Recognize the achievements along the way, no matter how small they may seem. This helps build confidence and resilience, providing the encouragement needed to tackle future challenges.

Interactive Element: Growth Mindset Reflection Exercise

Take a moment to think about a recent challenge you faced. Write down how you initially felt about it and what you learned through the experience. Consider how you can apply this learning to future situations. Reflecting on these moments can shift your perspective and strengthen your growth mindset, turning obstacles into opportunities for personal development.

STRATEGIES FOR STRESS REDUCTION

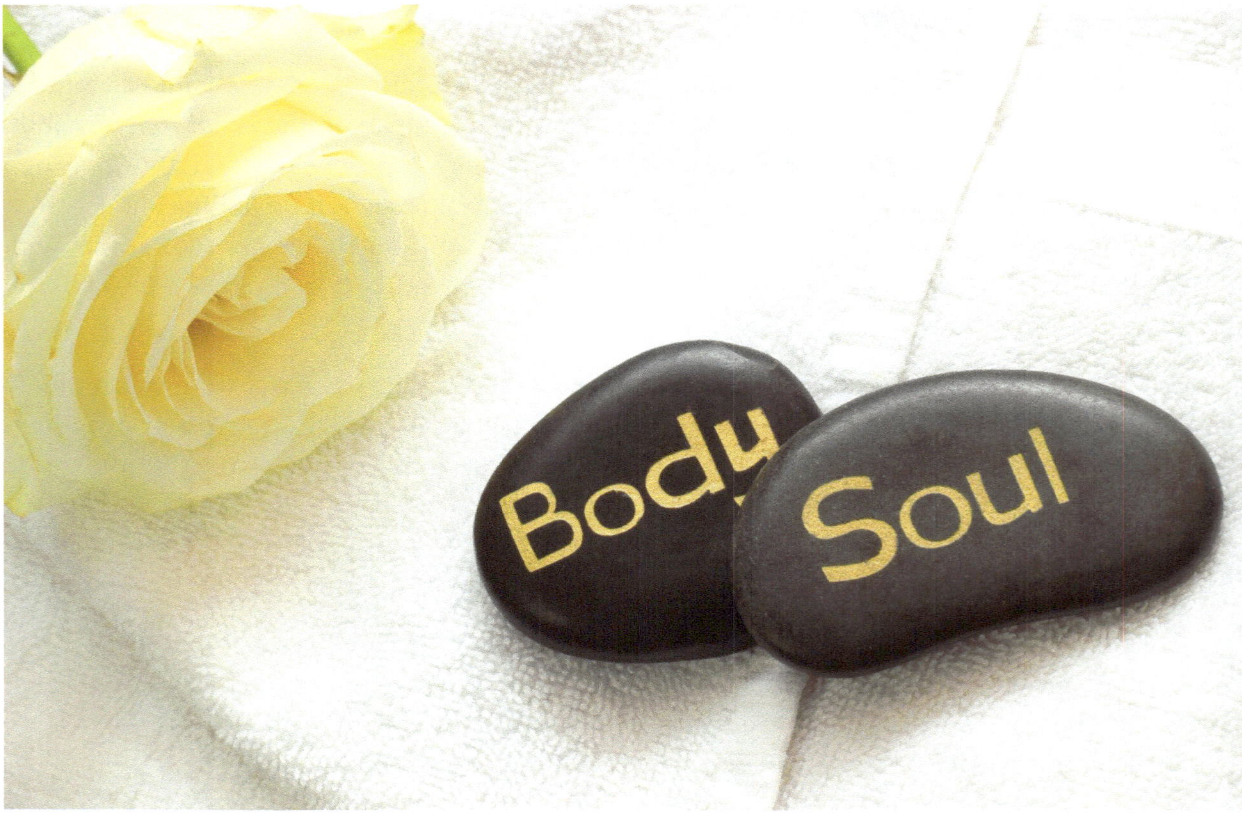

Stress has a way of creeping into our lives, sometimes without us even noticing until it's sitting heavily on our shoulders. For many adults, especially those with ADHD, identifying the sources of stress can be the first step toward managing it. Work-related pressure is a common culprit. Whether it's looming deadlines or the constant demand to multitask, work can often feel like a relentless treadmill, leaving you breathless and exhausted. Relationship dynamics also play a significant role. Misunderstandings, unspoken expectations, or conflicts with loved ones can create emotional turbulence that feels hard to navigate. Then there are the environmental triggers—the overflowing inbox, the cluttered desk, or even the noise of the city—that can amplify stress without you realizing it.

Recognizing these patterns and how they manifest in your body and mind is crucial. Do you notice tension in your shoulders when a deadline approaches? Or perhaps you feel a knot in your stomach after a disagreement with a partner? These physical and emotional cues are your body's way of signaling stress, and they can be invaluable in pinpointing your unique stressors.

Once you've identified these stressors, it's time to explore techniques that can help alleviate them. Progressive muscle relaxation is a method I find particularly helpful. It involves tensing and then slowly releasing each muscle group in your body, starting from your toes and working your way up. This technique not only provides immediate relief but also trains your body to recognize and counteract tension. Meditation and breathing exercises offer long-term benefits for stress management. Taking just a few minutes each day to focus on your breath can ground you, bringing a sense of calm and clarity that extends beyond the meditation session.

Engaging in hobbies and creative outlets is another powerful way to manage stress. Whether it's painting, playing music, or gardening, losing yourself in an activity you love can act as a reset button, allowing you to step back from your stressors and gain perspective.

Building a stress-resilient lifestyle involves more than just managing stress when it appears. It's about creating a foundation that supports overall well-being, making it easier to handle stress when it comes. Establishing a routine that balances work and leisure is essential. This might mean setting boundaries around your work hours or ensuring you make time for activities that recharge you. Building a support network is equally important. Having friends, family, or a community you can lean on provides both emotional and practical assistance. Sometimes, just knowing someone is there to listen can make all the difference.

Beyond personal connections, don't hesitate to utilize professional resources. Counseling and therapy can offer valuable insights and coping strategies tailored to your needs. Many workplaces also offer employee assistance programs, which provide support for work-related stress and other personal issues.

Recognizing when to seek professional help is crucial. If you find that stress is overwhelming or interfering with your daily life, reaching out to a therapist or counselor can be a positive step. They can provide a safe space to explore your stressors and develop strategies for coping. Remember, asking for help isn't a sign of weakness; it's a step toward taking control of your well-being. Whether it's through one-on-one sessions or group therapy, professional support can offer guidance, helping you navigate the complexities of stress with more confidence and clarity.

Stress may be an inevitable part of life, but with the right tools and support, it doesn't have to dictate your experience. Embrace the opportunity to create a lifestyle that supports you, allowing you to face stress with resilience and ease.

Interactive Element: Stress Mapping Exercise

Take a moment to create a stress map. On a piece of paper, list your common stressors, whether they're related to work, relationships, or daily life. Next to each stressor, note any physical or emotional symptoms you experience. This exercise will help you visualize your stress landscape, making it easier to identify patterns and develop targeted strategies for managing them. By understanding your stressors, you can take proactive steps to reduce their impact, paving the way for a more balanced and fulfilling life.

OVERCOMING SETBACKS WITH GRACE

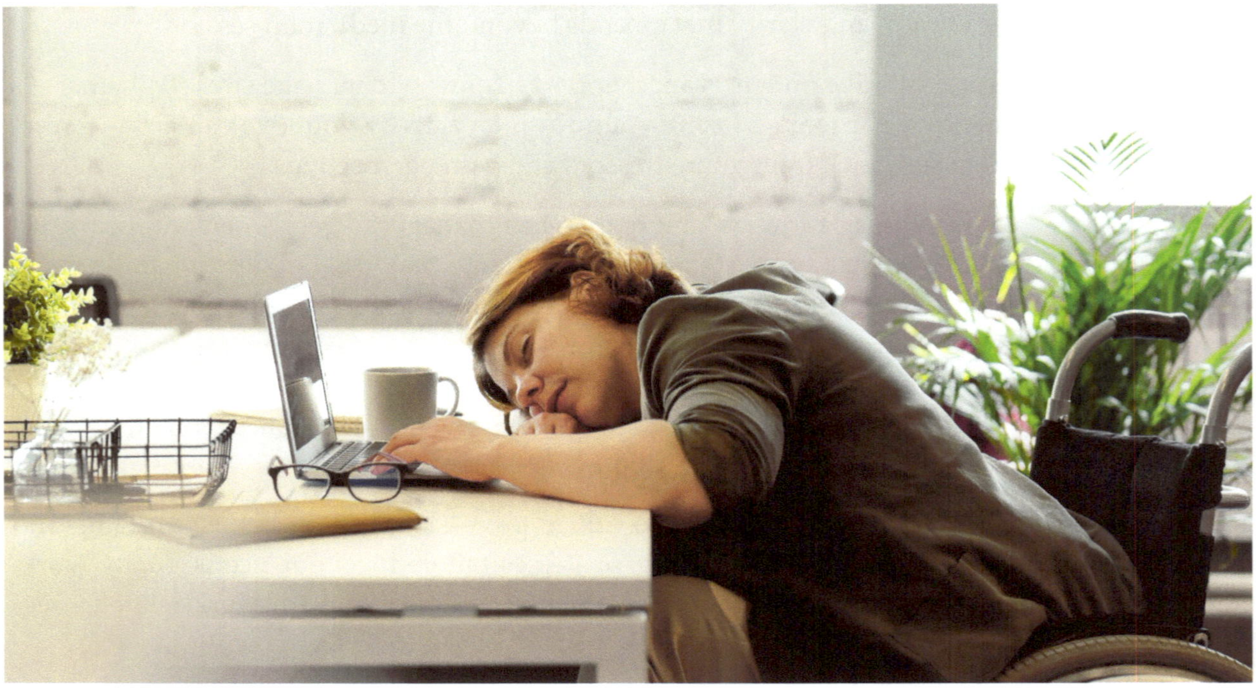

We've all been there—standing in the aftermath of a setback, feeling like we've just been knocked off a horse. There's that initial sting of disappointment and the whisper of doubt that creeps in, asking if we're cut out for this at all. But here's the thing: setbacks don't have to be roadblocks. They can be stepping stones if we choose to see them that way. Think of them as the universe's way of handing you a pop quiz. Instead of focusing on the fact that you tripped, take a closer look at the path. Analyze what went wrong. Was it a misjudgment of timing? Maybe a gap in preparation or resources? By dissecting these moments, you uncover the lessons hidden within. Each setback offers insights, like clues on a treasure map, guiding you toward change and improvement. Embrace these moments as opportunities to recalibrate and refine your approach. It's not about the fall; it's about how you rise after it.

Developing coping strategies is key—like having a toolkit ready for when those inevitable setbacks occur. Mindfulness is a powerful ally in these times. It keeps you grounded and present, helping you to focus on the here and now rather than spiraling into what-ifs. Take a few deep breaths, center yourself, and let the fog of disappointment clear. This clarity opens up space for problem-solving exercises. Break down the issue into smaller, manageable parts and tackle them one by one. This method not only provides direction but also helps in regaining control over the situation. Seeing each part separately can make the problem seem less daunting and more approachable, turning what felt like a mountain into a series of small hills. Each hill you climb brings you closer to the peak, building confidence and resilience along the way.

Staying motivated in the face of setbacks can feel like trying to light a match in a storm. It's challenging but not impossible. One way to keep the fire burning is by setting small, incremental goals. These are tiny victories that help rebuild momentum and keep you moving forward. They act as reminders that progress is happening, even if it feels slow. Visualization is another powerful tool. Picture your long-term success vividly. Imagine what it looks like, feels like, and even smells like. Let that vision be your lighthouse, guiding you through the fog of doubt and uncertainty. Each small step you take is a step closer to that vision becoming a reality. This focus not only keeps you motivated but also reinforces your commitment to your goals.

Learning from role models who have faced adversity and triumphed can be incredibly inspiring. Their stories of resilience and determination serve as reminders that setbacks are not the end—they're part of the narrative. Dive into biographies or listen to interviews of public figures who have been through similar struggles. Their journeys often reveal that failure is not the opposite of success but a part of it. Personal mentors can also be invaluable. Having someone who believes in you and offers guidance can provide the support you need to navigate rough patches. They can offer insights and encouragement that help you see beyond the immediate setback, reinforcing the belief that you can overcome it.

Remember, setbacks are not failures. They're invitations to learn, adapt, and grow. Each time you get back up, you build resilience and strength. It's about embracing the process, trusting that with each step forward, you're becoming stronger and more equipped to handle whatever comes your way. So, when you stumble, take a deep breath, dust yourself off, and keep moving. The path may not always be smooth, but it's yours to walk, and each step is bringing you closer to where you want to be.

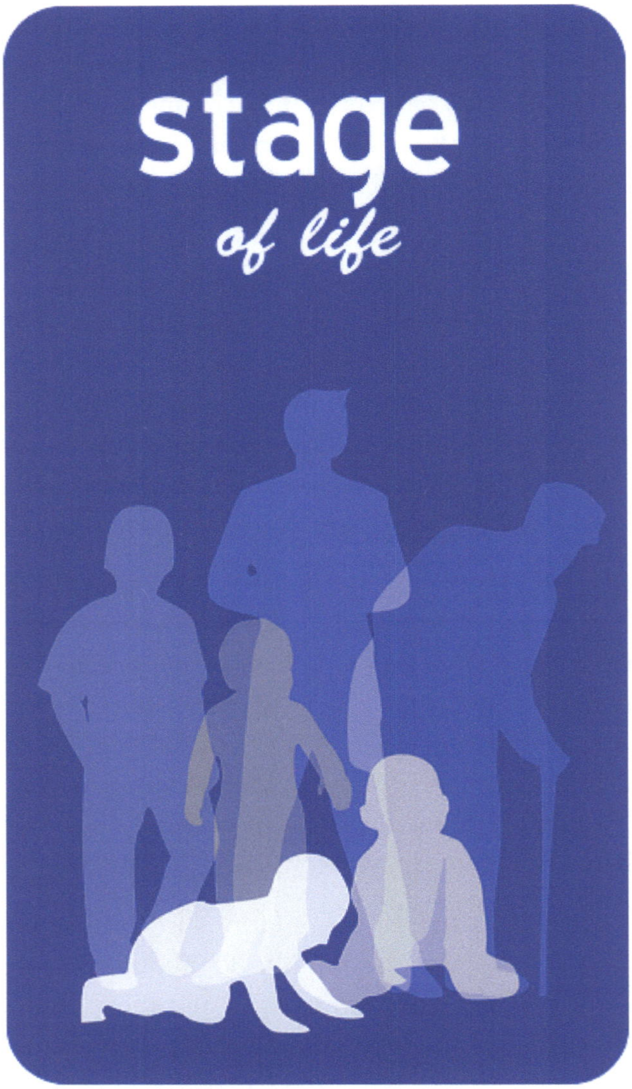

Life transitions can feel like standing on the edge of a cliff, looking out over an unknown landscape, unsure of what lies beyond. Whether it's a career change, the beginning or end of a relationship, or any significant life event, these shifts often come with a whirlwind of emotions. They can bring excitement and fear, hope and uncertainty, all mixed into a potent cocktail that leaves you both thrilled and terrified at once. The emotional rollercoaster that accompanies these changes is a natural response to stepping into the unfamiliar. It's like being on a ride that takes you up with anticipation and down into valleys of doubt. Each turn can be exhilarating or nerve-wracking, testing your resilience and adaptability.

Preparing for transitions is a bit like packing for a long journey, ensuring you have everything you need to navigate whatever may come. Creating a transition plan with actionable steps can be invaluable. Break down the process into manageable chunks, setting realistic expectations and timelines. This plan becomes your roadmap, guiding you through the fog of change. It's important to be flexible, allowing for detours and adjustments as needed. Life rarely follows a straight path, and being open to re-routing can help ease the stress of the transition.

Setting realistic expectations also means giving yourself grace—understanding that it's okay not to have everything figured out immediately. Timelines can be guidelines, not rigid deadlines, allowing you to progress at a pace that feels comfortable.

Adjusting to new roles and environments is akin to learning to dance with a new partner. It requires a mix of patience, adaptability, and willingness to learn. Building new routines can establish a sense of stability amidst the chaos of change. These routines act as anchors, providing a sense of normalcy and control in an otherwise fluid situation.

It's also crucial to seek out new opportunities for growth and learning. Change often opens doors to experiences and perspectives that were previously unavailable. Embrace these opportunities as chances to expand your horizons, learn new skills, or deepen your understanding of yourself and the world around you. This proactive approach not only aids in adaptation but also enriches your life, turning transitions into periods of growth and discovery.

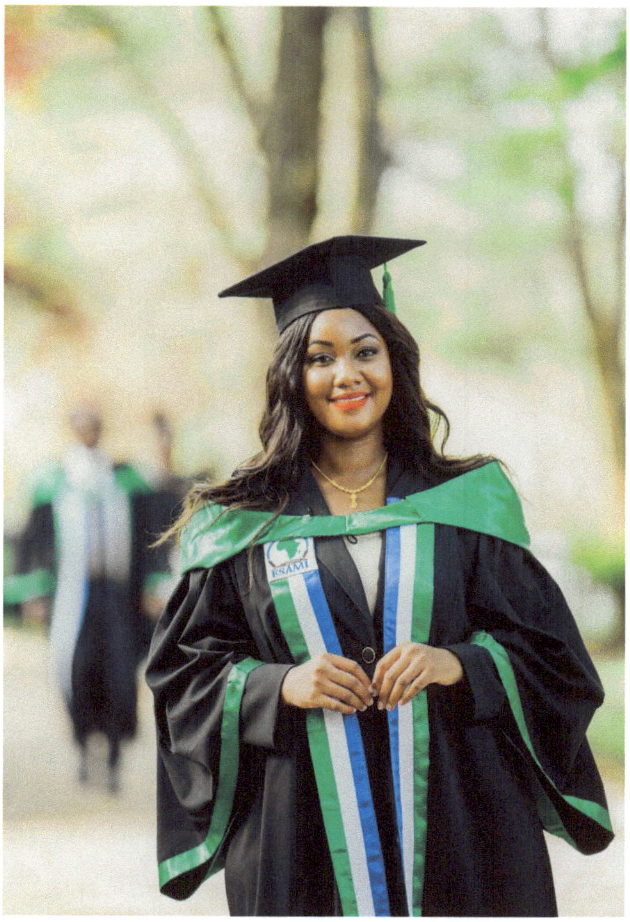

Celebrating personal growth through transitions is about recognizing the progress you've made along the way. Each milestone, no matter how small, is a testament to your resilience and adaptability. Reflect on these achievements, acknowledging the strength it took to get through the tough parts. It's easy to focus on what still needs to be done, but taking time to celebrate what you've accomplished is equally important. This reflection fosters a sense of gratitude and pride, reinforcing the idea that you are capable of navigating whatever life throws your way. It's about appreciating the journey, recognizing the lessons learned, and building confidence for future challenges.

Interactive Element: Transition Reflection Exercise

Take a moment to reflect on a recent transition you've experienced. Write down the challenges you faced and the strategies that helped you overcome them. List any milestones or achievements you reached along the way, and consider how they've contributed to your personal growth. This exercise can provide clarity, helping you see the progress you've made and reinforcing your ability to handle change.

Though daunting, transitions are a natural part of life. They shape who we are and who we become, teaching us resilience, adaptability, and the importance of staying open to new possibilities. As you navigate these changes, remember that each step forward is a step toward the person you're becoming. Embrace the process and trust in your ability to adapt and thrive. Next, we'll explore how fostering creativity and innovation can further enhance your ability to navigate life's complexities.

CHAPTER 11
CULTIVATING CREATIVITY AND INNOVATION

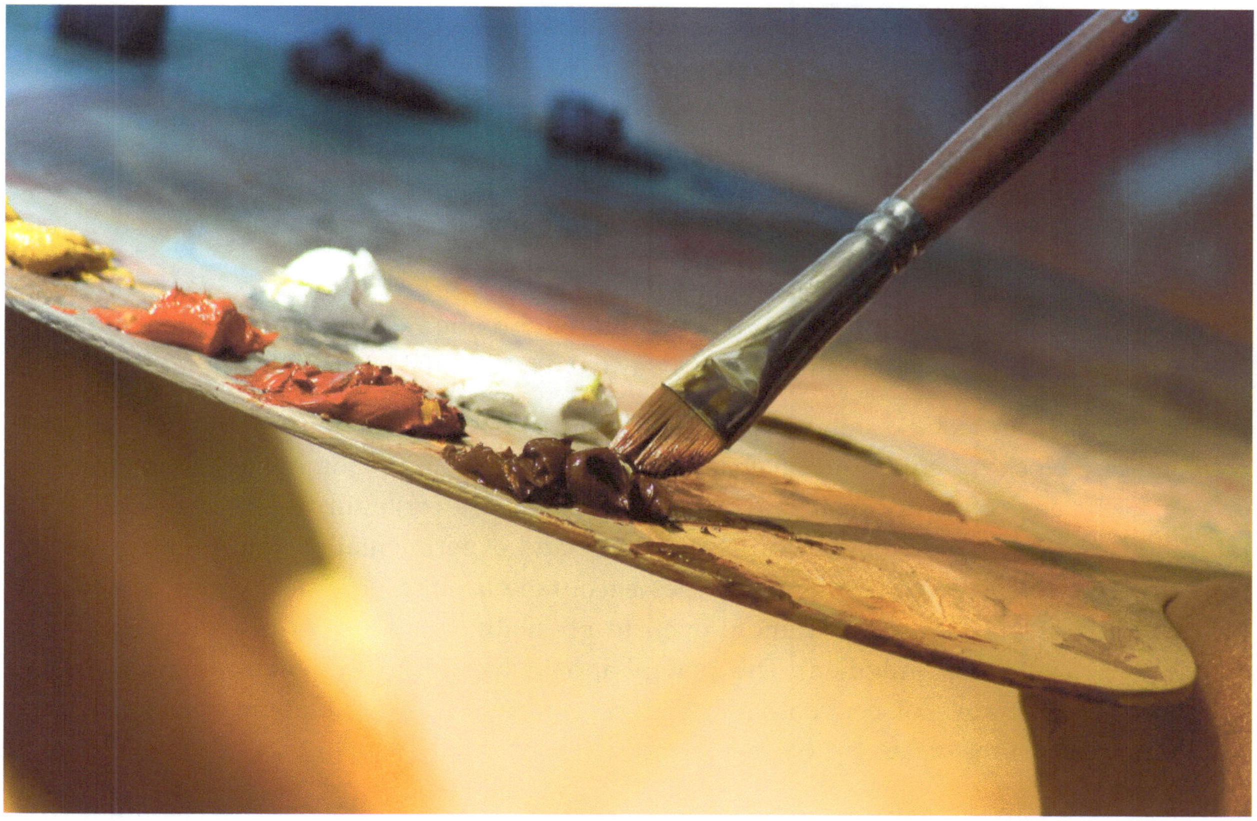

THERE WAS a time when I believed creativity was like a lightning bolt—rare, unpredictable, and entirely out of my control. It would strike at odd moments, often when I was least prepared to harness it. I'd be in the shower or drifting off to sleep, and suddenly, a brilliant idea would flash into my mind, only to disappear as quickly as it came. But then, I stumbled upon an approach that changed everything: seeing creativity not as a fleeting spark but as a skill that can be nurtured and developed. This perspective shifted my approach to problem-solving, teaching me that creativity doesn't just happen—it can be cultivated through practice, patience, and a willingness to view challenges from new angles.

Creative problem-solving is more than just coming up with new ideas; it's about approaching complex issues with a mindset that embraces innovation and lateral thinking. Conventional problem-solving often follows a linear path, sticking to tried-and-true methods that may not always yield the most effective results. In contrast, creative problem-solving invites us to think outside the box, exploring unconventional routes that might lead to unexpected solutions. Lateral thinking plays a central role in this process, encouraging us to step sideways from the usual path and consider alternatives that aren't immediately obvious. It's about seeing the world not as it is but as it could be and finding the connections between seemingly unrelated elements to create something entirely new.

Enhancing creativity isn't about waiting for inspiration to strike; it's about actively seeking opportunities to think differently. One effective strategy is to engage in brainstorming sessions where judgment is suspended, allowing ideas to flow freely without the constraints of immediate evaluation. This environment encourages bold thinking and the generation of a wide range of solutions, some of which may initially seem far-fetched but could hold the seeds of innovation. Another powerful tool is the SCAMPER technique, which stands for Substitute, Combine, Adapt, Modify, Put to another use, Eliminate, and Reverse. This method prompts us to apply these seven approaches to existing products or processes, sparking new ideas and perspectives.

For example, by considering how a product could be modified or combined with another, we might discover a novel solution that breaks away from traditional limitations.

Creative blocks can feel like hitting a wall, with ideas stalling and motivation waning. Overcoming these blocks often requires a change of scenery or mindset. Sometimes, simply moving to a different environment can inspire new perspectives, as fresh surroundings stimulate the mind and break the monotony. Incorporating play and experimentation into problem-solving can also reignite creativity, as these activities encourage a sense of curiosity and exploration. Like children at play, we become more open to possibilities, willing to take risks and make mistakes without fear of judgment. This playful approach can lead to breakthroughs, as it frees us from the constraints of conventional thinking and allows us to embrace the unexpected twists and turns of the creative process.

Applying creativity to real-world challenges involves translating imaginative solutions into practical applications that address everyday problems. For example, developing novel marketing strategies can set a small business apart from its competitors. By leveraging creative problem-solving techniques, business owners can identify unique selling points and craft campaigns that resonate with target audiences in fresh and engaging ways. In the workplace, designing unique solutions for efficiency can lead to significant improvements in productivity and morale. By encouraging employees to think creatively about their tasks and responsibilities, organizations can foster an environment where innovation thrives and new ideas are not only welcomed but celebrated.

Interactive Element: Creativity Journal

Set aside time each day to jot down three things that sparked your curiosity or made you think differently. This could be anything from a conversation with a friend to a piece of art that caught your eye. Reflect on these moments and consider how they might inform your approach to a current challenge. Keep this journal as a resource to revisit and draw inspiration from when you need a creative boost.

TURNING IDEAS INTO ACTION

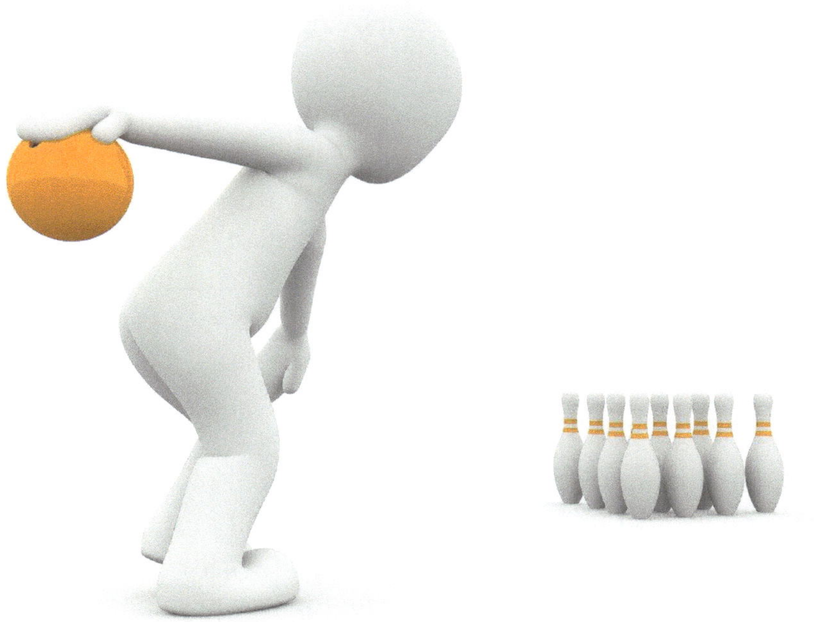

Taking a creative idea and transforming it into a tangible project feels like bringing a dream to life. It's not just about having a spark of inspiration but about crafting that raw idea into something real and impactful. The first step in this process is developing a clear vision and purpose for your project. Think about what you want to achieve and why it matters. This clarity acts as your North Star, guiding every decision you make along the way. Once the vision is set, create a step-by-step action plan. Break down the project into smaller, manageable tasks and set achievable milestones. These milestones are like checkpoints that keep you on track and motivated, allowing you to celebrate small victories along the way.

When it comes to planning and executing creative projects, organization is your best friend. Tools like Trello or Asana can be incredibly helpful in keeping everything organized. They allow you to map out each phase of your project, assign tasks, and track progress. Setting realistic timelines is crucial. It's easy to get caught up in the excitement of a new idea, but rushing can lead to burnout or overlooked details. Allocate resources wisely, whether it's time, money, or manpower. Be honest about what you can realistically achieve with the resources you have. This planning stage is where your idea starts to take shape, moving from abstract to concrete.

Execution, however, can present its own set of challenges. Perfectionism often rears its head, whispering that your work isn't good enough. Fear of failure can paralyze you, making it tempting to abandon the project altogether. But remember, perfection is an illusion. Progress is what counts. Adjust your plans when necessary—accept feedback, embrace unforeseen issues, and adapt. Flexibility is key. Plans are not set in stone; they are meant to evolve as your project unfolds. This adaptability allows you to keep moving forward, even when things don't go exactly as expected.

Once your project is complete, it's time to share it with the world. This is both exhilarating and nerve-wracking, but it's an important step that shouldn't be skipped. Host a showcase event, whether online or in person, to present your work to a broader audience. Create an online portfolio to document your creative journey. Utilize social media platforms to increase visibility and engagement with your project. Sharing your work not only validates your efforts but also opens doors to new opportunities and collaborations. It allows others to see the value of your creativity, fostering connections and potentially leading to new projects.

Oh right Interactive Element: Project Planning Template

Create a project planning template that outlines your vision, purpose, and step-by-step action plan. Include sections for timelines, resources, and potential obstacles. Use this template as a roadmap to guide your project from concept to completion. Revisit and revise it as needed, ensuring it remains aligned with your evolving goals and circumstances.

COLLABORATIVE CREATIVITY: WORKING WITH OTHERS

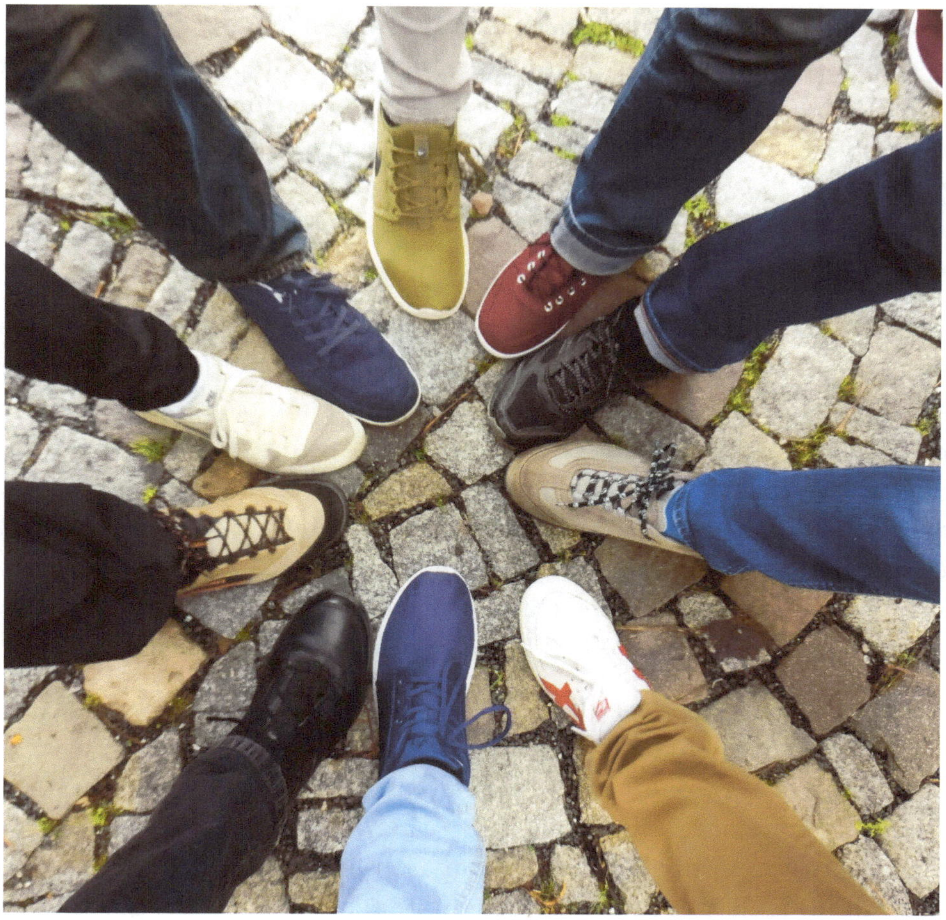

There's something truly magical about bringing together different minds around a table—whether literal or metaphorical—and watching ideas bounce off each other like sparks. I've experienced firsthand how collaboration fuels creativity, transforming simple thoughts into groundbreaking innovations. When you work with others, you're not just adding up ideas; you're creating a synergy where one person's insight can amplify another's, leading to more intricate and enriched solutions. This melting pot of perspectives challenges the status quo and pushes boundaries, resulting in solutions that one mind alone might never conjure. It's this diversity of thought—each person viewing the problem through their own unique lens—that often leads to the most creative and effective outcomes. Plus, having multiple brains tackling a problem means you can draw on a wider pool of experiences, skills, and expertise. It's like having a Swiss Army knife for problem-solving, each tool honed by different hands, ready to cut through complexity with ease.

Building an effective creative team is akin to assembling a dream cast for a movie, with each member bringing something special to the storyline. Start by identifying complementary skills and strengths within the group. You want a mix of talents and viewpoints—someone who's detail-oriented might catch the things the big-picture thinker misses, while the strategist can map out the plan inspired by the visionary's ideas. Clear roles and responsibilities are crucial, as they provide structure and prevent the chaos that can sometimes come with creativity. Everyone should know their part in the bigger picture, like pieces of a puzzle fitting together to create a coherent image. It's also important to foster an open and inclusive team culture where each voice is valued and encouraged. This environment not only nurtures creativity but also ensures that members feel safe to express their thoughts without fear of judgment or dismissal. Inclusivity breeds innovation, as it brings hidden ideas to light and keeps the creative engine running smoothly.

Facilitating effective collaboration requires more than just putting people in a room together. It's about creating an ecosystem where ideas can flourish and evolve. Tools like Google Workspace or Miro can be invaluable here, allowing for seamless collaboration regardless of location. These platforms offer real-time sharing and feedback, enabling teams to brainstorm and refine ideas collectively. Open dialogue is key, and constructive criticism should be viewed as a stepping stone rather than a stumbling block. Encourage team members to voice their thoughts openly, fostering a culture where feedback is welcomed and used to enhance the collective output. This dynamic exchange not only enriches the creative process but also strengthens the team's ability to tackle challenges head-on, armed with a blend of perspectives and insights.

Navigating group dynamics can feel like walking a tightrope, where balance is essential to maintain harmony. Sometimes, you'll encounter dominant voices that overpower quieter ones, and it's crucial to ensure everyone's ideas are heard and considered. Techniques such as round-robin discussions or anonymous idea submissions can help balance these dynamics, giving each team member an equal opportunity to contribute. Conflict, while often seen as a negative, can actually be a catalyst for deeper understanding and innovation if managed constructively. It's important to approach disagreements with a mindset focused on resolution rather than blame. Encourage open discussions about differing viewpoints, aiming to find common ground or even merge ideas into something stronger. This approach not only resolves conflicts but also strengthens the team's cohesion and resilience.

Interactive Element: Team Dynamics Exercise

Try this: In your next team meeting, start with a round-robin session in which everyone shares one idea or thought. Then, follow up with a group discussion on how these ideas can be integrated or improved. Use a tool like Miro to visually map out the discussion, highlighting connections and new insights. This exercise not only helps balance group dynamics but also fosters a deeper appreciation for each team member's unique contributions.

INNOVATING WITH PURPOSE

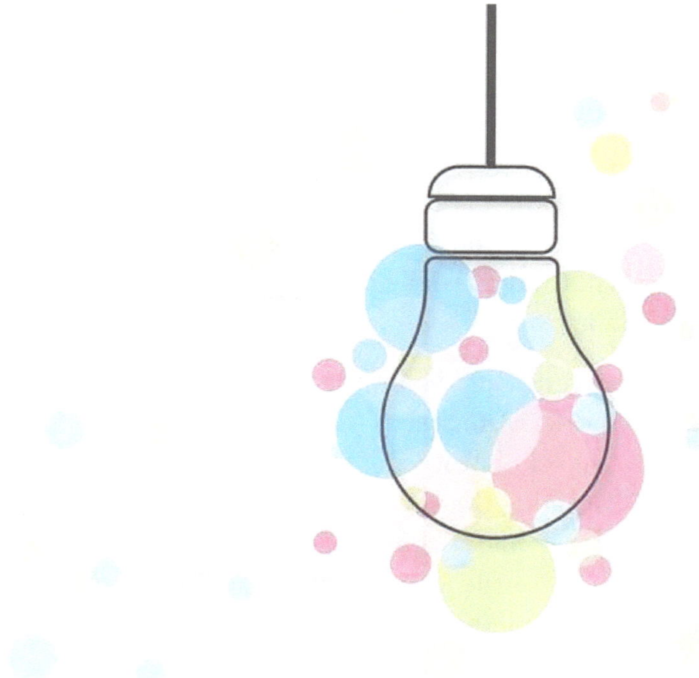

Bringing innovation into our lives isn't just about creating new gadgets or flashy technologies. It's about making meaningful changes that resonate with our values and address genuine needs. Think about the problems that make you pause—those societal issues you wish you could solve, or personal challenges that keep you up at night. Innovation with purpose means aligning our creative efforts with personal beliefs and the wider world's needs. This alignment ensures that what we create has depth and significance, addressing real-world problems while also satisfying our inner drive for meaning.

When innovation is guided by purpose, it not only solves problems but also fosters a sense of fulfillment, knowing that our work contributes positively to society. Sustainability and ethics must be at the heart of purposeful innovation. As we develop new ideas, it's crucial to consider their long-term impact on the environment and society. This means designing solutions that are not only effective but also sustainable and ethical, ensuring that our innovations do not compromise the well-being of future generations. By integrating these considerations into our creative processes, we can create solutions that are both innovative and responsible, benefiting both people and the planet.

To innovate with purpose, you first need to identify areas where your skills and passions intersect with societal demands. Think about what excites you and where you can make a difference. Conducting market research is a practical starting point. This involves exploring existing gaps in products or services and considering how your unique insights could fill those voids. Unmet needs are often the breeding ground for impactful innovation, providing opportunities to create solutions that truly resonate with people. By understanding these gaps, you can align your efforts with areas that not only interest you but also serve a broader purpose.

Exploring the intersection of personal interests and societal demands involves looking at current trends and societal shifts. Consider how your expertise or passion can address emerging challenges, such as climate change or mental health. This alignment ensures that your innovation is both personally fulfilling and socially relevant, allowing you to contribute to causes that matter to you and your community. By focusing on these intersections, you can identify opportunities where your skills and passions can make a meaningful impact, driving innovation that is both purposeful and impactful.

Technology can be a powerful ally in amplifying the impact of purposeful innovation. Emerging technologies, like Artificial Intelligence (AI) and the Internet of Things (IoT), have the potential to revolutionize how we solve problems. AI, for example, can analyze vast amounts of data to uncover patterns and insights that humans might miss, enabling us to develop more effective solutions. IoT, on the other hand, connects devices and systems, allowing for real-time monitoring and control, which can lead to more efficient and innovative solutions. By leveraging these technologies, we can enhance the reach and effectiveness of our innovations, transforming ideas into impactful realities.

Digital platforms also play a crucial role in reaching wider audiences. They provide a space to share our innovations, gather feedback, and build a community around our ideas. By developing a strong online presence, we can connect with like-minded individuals and potential collaborators, amplifying the impact of our work and driving further innovation. These platforms also offer opportunities to gather feedback from users, helping us refine our ideas and ensure that they meet the needs of those they are intended to serve. By embracing technology, we can extend the reach of our innovations, making a positive impact on a global scale.

Assessing the impact of our innovations is key to gauging their effectiveness and ensuring they meet their objectives. Establishing clear metrics for success allows us to objectively evaluate our projects, identifying what excels and what requires adjustments. These metrics might range from quantitative data like sales figures and user engagement to qualitative insights such as customer satisfaction or the broader social impact. Implementing these metrics from the start enables us to monitor progress and fine-tune our innovations accordingly.

Feedback from stakeholders and end-users plays a critical role in this assessment process, offering unique perspectives on how our innovations are received and interacted with. This feedback loop not only highlights areas for enhancement but also opens up avenues for further innovation, ensuring our solutions stay relevant and impactful. By fostering a collaborative environment, stakeholders' insights contribute to the ongoing refinement of our projects, aligning them more closely with user needs and expectations. Through continuous measurement and adjustment, we can maintain the relevance and efficacy of our innovations, thereby maximizing their positive contribution to society.

CONCLUSION

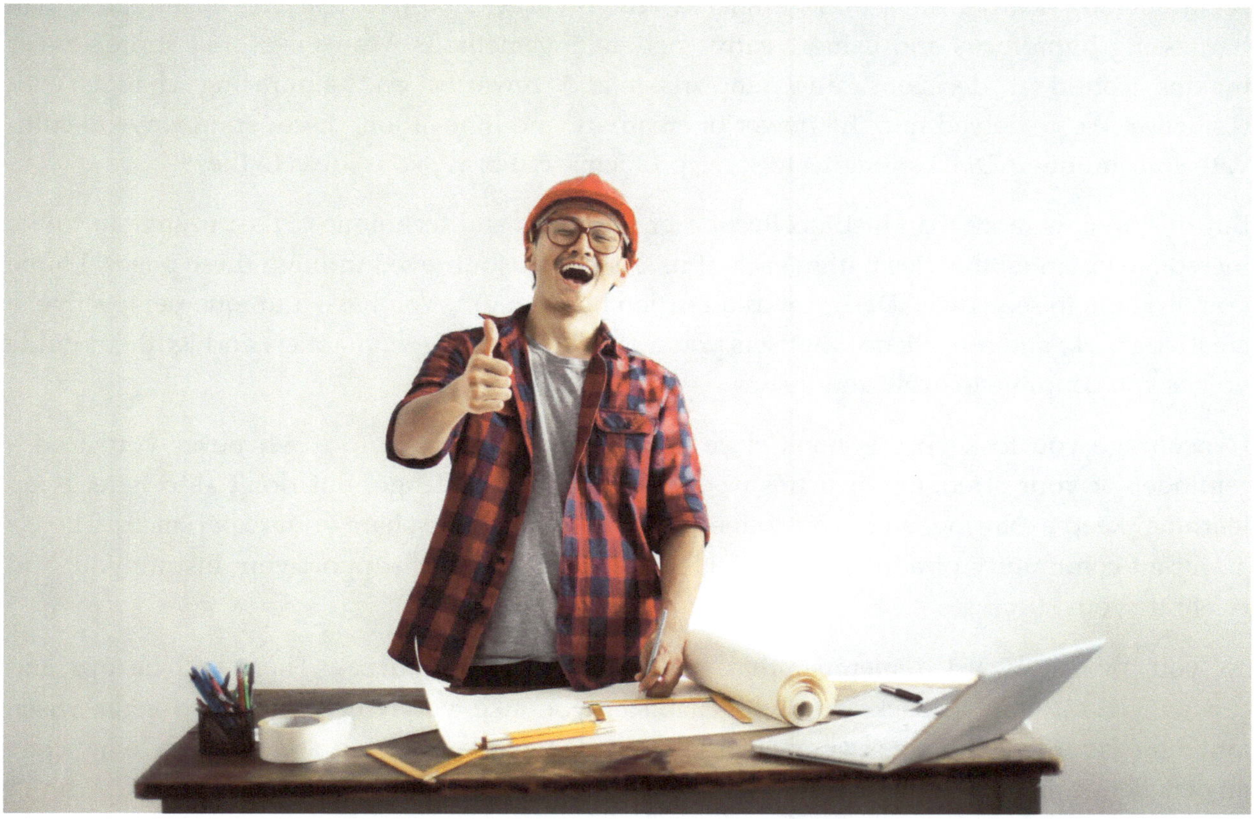

As we approach the end of our journey together, I want to take a moment to reflect. When I first set out to write this book, my goal was to create a resource that would empower adults with ADHD to embrace their unique strengths and thrive in all aspects of life. I wanted to share my own experiences—both the triumphs and the challenges—to show you that you're not alone in this journey.

Throughout these pages, we've explored the many facets of living with ADHD. We've delved into the importance of understanding and accepting your neurodiversity, recognizing that ADHD isn't a limitation but rather a different way of thinking and experiencing the world. We've discovered strategies for mastering time management, like the Pomodoro Technique and visual planners, to help you stay focused and productive. We've also tackled the emotional aspects of ADHD, learning techniques for enhancing emotional regulation, such as mindfulness practices and identifying triggers.

You've seen how nurturing relationships, both with yourself and others, is key to thriving with ADHD. We've discussed the art of clear communication, managing conflicts, and building a supportive community. We've also emphasized the importance of self-care and wellness, from creating personalized routines to understanding the impact of nutrition and exercise on your ADHD brain.

As a lifelong learner myself, I've shared my favorite adaptive learning techniques, like harnessing hyperfocus and using creative note-taking methods. We've explored strategies for making confident decisions, analyzing risks and rewards, and embracing change with resilience. We've delved into the power of creativity and innovation, discovering ways to cultivate your unique ADHD strengths to solve problems and bring your ideas to life.

But this book is more than just a collection of strategies and techniques. It's a testament to the incredible potential that lies within each of us. As you've journeyed through these pages, I hope you've come to see your ADHD not as a burden but as a gift. You have a unique perspective, a creative spark, and a resilience that sets you apart. Embrace these qualities, and let them guide you as you continue to grow and thrive.

I encourage you to keep this book close at hand, referring back to it whenever you need a reminder of your strengths or a fresh perspective on a challenge. But don't stop here. Keep learning, keep exploring, and keep connecting with others who share your experiences. There's a vibrant community of adults with ADHD out there, ready to support you, inspire you, and celebrate your successes.

As you move forward, remember that growth is a lifelong journey. There will be ups and downs, victories and setbacks. But with each step you take, you're becoming a stronger, wiser, and more confident version of yourself. You have the tools, knowledge, and strength to navigate any challenge that comes your way.

So, my friend, I invite you to step boldly into your future. Embrace your ADHD journey with curiosity, compassion, and a sense of adventure. You have so much to offer the world, and I can't wait to see the incredible things you'll achieve.

Thank you for allowing me to be a part of your journey. It's been an honor to share my story with you and to help you discover the extraordinary potential that lies within you. Remember, you are capable of amazing things. Never doubt your worth, your creativity, or your ability to make a difference.

Keep shining brightly, and know that I'm cheering you on every step of the way. Here's to the incredible journey ahead!

With gratitude and admiration, Jamaal Simmons

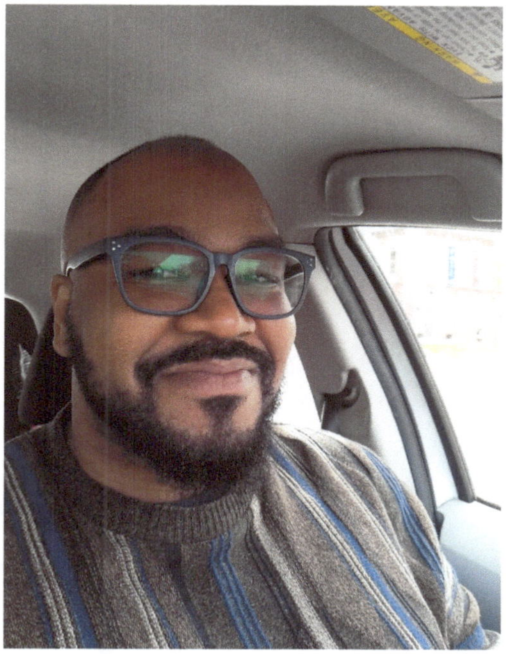

ACKNOWLEDGMENTS

I want to thank everyone who's helped support me and helped me on my journey here to write my first full-length book. Before this, I did five coloring books, and at some point, I would like to redo them and make them even better. However, I don't want to be a perfectionist either, so I will have to balance that at some point. I would love to thank my adoptive family, aka my family, for always being there for me And giving me the love, support, and guidance I needed. I would also like to thank my fiance, Michelle, for being so supportive of me and my ADHD moments. If it wasn't for her, I don't know if I would have written this book because she gave me some tough love about being focused, and she knows how I love chasing the next dopamine high instead of focusing! I would also like to thank my kids and my new stepkids. I appreciate their honesty And their ability to humble me.

I would also love to thank my mentors because I wouldn't have gotten this far without them, including my mental health mentor, Terri E. Johnson, and my real estate mentor, Jim Quimby. I'm so grateful they accepted me as their mentee whether they wanted to or not because it would happen anyway. I would also like to thank my friends who have been there for me for a long time and even my new friends who have started to be there for me. It's been a long journey, and acknowledging how I've been helped is a humbling honor. I'm smiling as I write this down, as I see the faces of all those who have helped me, and I hope to help them back as well. Even though I tend to be a lone wolf, I fully recognize that we're all in this together, and this is my tribe. These are my people. And I'm so grateful for them.

REVIEW REQUEST

Now that you've learned how to understand and embrace ADHD, it's time to share your new knowledge and help others find the same support. By leaving your honest review of this book on Amazon, you'll show other adults with ADHD, parents of ADHD children, and therapy clients where they can find the guidance they need. Your review will help them discover how to turn ADHD challenges into strengths and unlock their full potential.

Thank you for being part of this journey. The power of ADHD Life Skills 101 grows when we share what we've learned—and you're helping me do just that.

Click here to leave your review on Amazon.

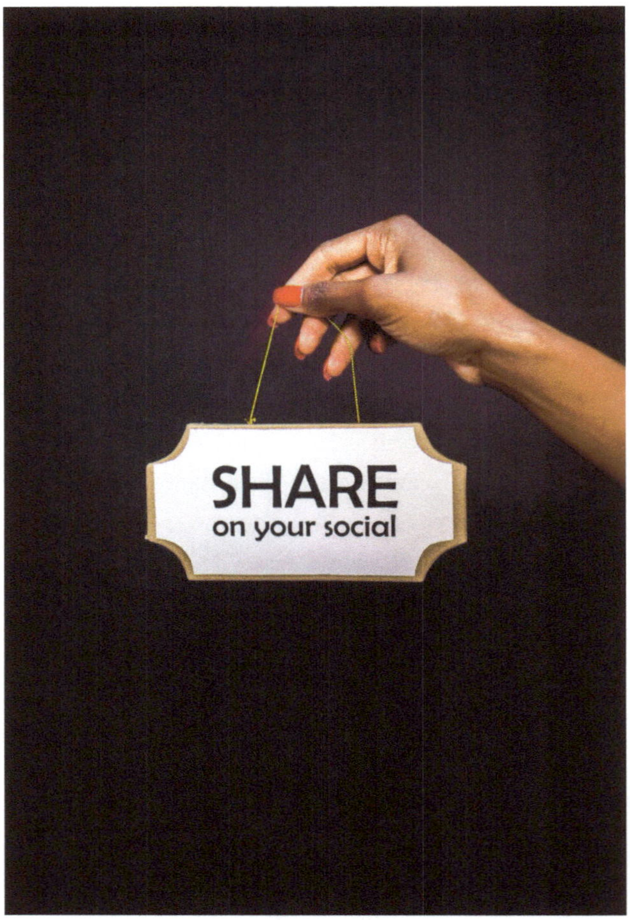

Social Media

Website: https://smhllc.squarespace.com

Link Tree: https://linktr.ee/SMHLLC

Instagram: https://www.instagram.com/smhllc/

LinkedIn: https://www.linkedin.com/in/smhllc/

Twitter: https://twitter.com/IoriShakor

Facebook: https://www.facebook.com/SimmonsMHLLC

Yelp: https://www.yelp.com/biz/simmons-mental-health-loch-raven

Youtube: www.youtube.com/@JamaalSpublishing

Twitch: twitch.tv/iorishakor

Psychology Today: https://www.psychologytoday.com/us/therapists/jamaal-simmons-towson-md/870507

Google Play Apps: https://play.google.com/store/apps/developer?id=Jamaal+S.+Publishing

TikTok: www.tiktok.com/@iori_shakor

Creator Spring: https://jamaalspublishing.creator-spring.com/

Link Tree: https://linktr.ee/SMHLLC

Link to Terri E. Johnson's Children's Book:

https://www.etsy.com/shop/PersistenceistheWAY

REFERENCES

- *Understanding Cultural Perspectives on Neurodiversity* https://www.urevolution.com/blogs/magazine/understanding-cultural-perspectives-on-neurodiversity?srsltid=AfmBOopXzQjFN2vP_6vc74zN4r7qbBh-30QXppjq7eGrkv4nNYuylPG4
- *Creativity in ADHD: Goal-Directed Motivation and Domain ...* https://pmc.ncbi.nlm.nih.gov/articles/PMC7543022/#:~:text=Results%3A%20Adults%20with%20ADHD%20reported,when%20competing%20for%20a%20bonus.
- *Gender differences in adult ADHD: Cognitive function ...* https://pmc.ncbi.nlm.nih.gov/articles/PMC7561166/#:~:text=Other%20studies%20suggest%20a%20gender,impulsivity%20%5B8%2C%2014%5D.
- *30 Famous People with ADHD Breaking the Stigma - Deepwrk* https://www.deepwrk.io/blog/famous-people-with-adhd#:~:text=While%20the%20modern%20concept%20of,%2C%20Walt%20Disney%2C%20John%20F.
- *Pomodoro Technique for ADHD Management* https://adhdandautismclinic.co.uk/unleashing-productivity-the-pomodoro-technique-for-adhd-management/#:~:text=The%20structured%20nature%20of%20the,perceiving%20and%20estimating%20time%20accurately.
- *Choosing the Best Planner for an ADHD Brain* https://www.erincondren.com/inspiration-center-best-planner-adhd?srsltid=AfmBOoqUT2T3xdhEgdLA0wVXKPlAlo1TwQu0MKtsjN9Mo4yd23UeK3RI
- *6 Online ADHD Management Tools for Adults - ADDA* https://add.org/adhd-tools-for-adults/
- *How to Use the 2-Minute Rule to Beat Procrastination* https://www.verywellmind.com/use-the-2-minute-rule-to-beat-procrastination-8720928
- *Mindfulness Meditation Training for Attention-Deficit/ ...* https://pmc.ncbi.nlm.nih.gov/articles/PMC4403871/
- *Taming Emotional Triggers with an ADHD Brain* https://drsharonsaline.com/2022/03/taming-emotional-triggers-with-an-adhd-brain-how-to-understand-big-feelings-and-respond-differently/
- *ADHD and Self-Compassion - CHADD* https://chadd.org/attention-article/adhd-and-self-compassion/#:~:text=Dr.,%2C%20optimism%2C%20and%20social%20connectedness.
- *Building Resilience in ADHD through Cognitive Flexibility* https://effectiveeffortconsulting.com/building-resilience-how-cognitive-flexibility-and-emotional-regulation-empower-adhd-individuals/
- *Unveiling Effective ADHD Communication Strategies* https://justmind.org/adhd-communication-strategies/
- *Conflict Resolution: A Skills Guide for ADHD Families and ...* https://www.additudemag.com/slideshows/conflict-resolution-skills-family-relationships-adhd/?srsltid=AfmBOooUb_Lflqf4axQV9zJ1j0rFV3B6kndZiuY6RZlsAP_yQA8pBciZ
- *How ADHD Influences Your Sex Life and Intimate ...* https://www.psychologytoday.com/us/blog/sex-esteem/202210/how-adhd-influences-your-sex-life-and-intimate-relationships
- *ADHD support groups: Benefits, options, and more* https://www.medicalnewstoday.com/articles/adhd-support-groups
- *An honest review of the top budgeting apps for people with ...* https://blog.rulemoney.co.uk/a-rundown-of-the-top-budgeting-apps-for-people-with-adhd/
- *ADHD Money Management: Financial Success And Stability* https://add.org/adhd-friendly-financial-management-yes-and-its-not-what-you-think/
- *Managing Money and ADHD: Expenses and Goals* https://chadd.org/for-adults/managing-money-and-adhd-expenses-and-goals/
- *ADHD Money Management: Financial Success And Stability* https://add.org/adhd-friendly-financial-management-yes-and-its-not-what-you-think/
- *StrengthsFinder 2.0* https://www.gallup.com/cliftonstrengths/en/254033/strengthsfinder.aspx
- *The ADHD-marketing connection: how neurodiversity drives ...* https://startupsmagazine.co.uk/article-adhd-

marketing-connection-how-neurodiversity-drives-success-industry-0#:~:text=People%20with%20ADHD%20often%20have,creativity%20and%20adaptability%20are%20essential.

- *15 Tips for Networking with ADHD (Challenges & Strategies)* https://adhdspecialist.com/post/networking-when-you-have-adhd
- *Overcoming Imposter Syndrome with ADHD* https://www.adhdcentre.co.uk/overcoming-imposter-syndrome-with-adhd/#:~:text=Embracing%20self%2Dcompassion%2C%20challenging%20negative,in%20all%20aspects%20of%20life.
- *Strategies for Adults Living With ADHD* https://advancedpsychiatryassociates.com/resources/blog/strategies-for-adults-living-with-adhd
- *ADHD Diet For Adults: Foods to Eat and Avoid - ADDA* https://add.org/adhd-diet/
- *What's the Best Exercise to Manage ADHD Symptoms?* https://www.webmd.com/add-adhd/exercise-manage-adhd-symptoms
- *Digital Detox for ADHD Brains: How to Limit Social Media, Texts* https://www.additudemag.com/digital-detox-social-media-adhd/
- *Tips for Managing Adult ADHD* https://www.helpguide.org/mental-health/adhd/managing-adult-adhd
- *Hyperfocus Symptoms: The Good, the Bad, and the Ugly* https://www.additudemag.com/hyperfocus-symptoms-positives-negatives-strategies/?srsltid=AfmBOoqPjqTIglBJC4t-2JRFw85swg_814xEE9P-2tYNH-okW4W2il7y
- *5 Strategies for Taking Better Notes for Students with ADHD* https://jamworks.com/news/5-strategies-taking-better-notes-students-adhd/#:~:text=Students%20with%20ADHD%20might%20benefit,and%20active%20note%20taking%20experience.
- *Supporting Success: Setting Appropriate IEP Goals for ADHD* https://everydayspeech.com/blog-posts/general/supporting-success-setting-appropriate-iep-goals-for-adhd/#:~:text=The%20SMART%20goal%20framework%20is,by%20providing%20clarity%20and%20structure.
- *ADHD and Decision Making: Symptoms, Tips, and More* https://psychcentral.com/adhd/adults-adhd-tips-to-make-good-decisions
- *How Does ADHD Intuition Differ from Neurotypical Intuition?* https://www.focusbear.io/blog-post/how-does-adhd-intuition-differ-from-neurotypical-intuition
- *15 Risk Management Tools and Techniques [2025]* https://www.simplilearn.com/risk-management-tools-article
- *An ADHD diagnosis in adulthood comes with challenges ...* https://www.apa.org/monitor/2023/03/adult-adhd-diagnosis
- *Understanding The Power of Mindset for ADHD Brains* https://www.addept.org/living-with-adult-add-adhd/growth-mindset-and-adult-add-adhd
- *ADHD Relaxation Techniques to Reduce Stress* https://www.additudemag.com/adhd-relaxation-techniques-to-reduce-stress/?srsltid=AfmBOoqdyFpr69kIP1khKn8nXgDF1lDRbqBY5wxJ_HgVlc38mNMjF-6u
- *How to Deal With Setbacks When Trying To Work With Your ...* https://marlacummins.com/how-to-deal-with-setbacks-when-working-with-your-adhd/#:~:text=get%20the%20support%20you%20need,have%20to%20re-peat%20the%20past.%E2%80%9D
- *Why Transitions Are Hard When You Have ADHD* https://adhdonline.com/articles/why-transitions-are-hard-when-you-have-adhd/
- *Creative Problem Solving: Solution Oriented ADHD Brains ...* https://www.additudemag.com/creative-problem-solving-adhd/
- *SCAMPER Technique Examples and Applications* https://www.designorate.com/scamper-technique-examples-and-applications/
- *Collaborate with Google Workspace and Miro* https://miro.com/integrations/google-workspace/
- *How Innovators Can Align Personal Values With Business ...* https://aaronhall.com/how-innovators-can-align-personal-values-with-business-decisions/

www.ingramcontent.com/pod-product-compliance
Lightning Source LLC
LaVergne TN
LVHW070936210926
848482LV00003B/257